INTERMITTENT

FOR WOMEN

THE **GOLDEN**

WINDOW FOR

WOMEN

The Essential Fast Metabolism
Diet Guide For Women To Lose
Weight Quickly and Effectively
Step-By-Step

ALISA BARR

Table of Contents

PART I

Chapter 1: Meal Planning 101

Sticking to a diet is something that is not the easiest in the world. When it comes down to it, we struggle to change up our diets on a whim. It might be that for the first few days, you are able to stick to it and make sure that you are only eating those foods that are better for you, but over time, you will get to a point where you feel the pressure to cave in. You might realize that sticking to your diet is difficult and think that stopping for a burger on your way home won't be too bad. You might think that figuring out lunch or dinner is too much of a hassle, or you realize that the foods that you have bought forgot a key ingredient that you needed for dinner.

The good news is, you have an easy fix. When you are able to figure out what you are making for yourself for your meals well in advance, you stop having to worry so much about the foods that you eat, what you do with them, and what you are going to reach for when it's time to eat. You will be able to change up what you are doing so that you can be certain that the meals that you are enjoying are good for you, and you won't have to worry so much about the stress that goes into it. Let's take a look at what you need to do to get started with meal planning so that you can begin to do so without having to think too much about it.

Make a Menu

First, before you do anything, make sure that you make a menu! This should be something that you do on your own, or you should sit down with your family to ask them what they prefer. If you can do this, you will be able to ensure that you've got a clear-cut plan. When you have a menu a week in advance, you save yourself time and money because you know that all of your meals will use ingredients that are similar, and you won't have to spend forever thinking about what you should make at any point in time.

Plan around Ads

When you do your menu, make it a point to glance through the weekly ads as well. Typically, you will find that there are plenty of deals that you can make use of that will save you money.

Go Meatless Once Per Week

A great thing to do that is highly recommended on the Mediterranean Diet is to have a day each week where you go meatless for dinner. By doing so, you will realize that you can actually cut costs and enjoy the foods more at the same time. It is a great way to get that additional fruit and veggie content into your day, and there are plenty of healthy options that are out there for you. You just have to commit to doing so. In the meal plans that you'll see below, you will notice that there will be a meatless day on Day 2 every week.

Use Ingredients That You Already Have On Hand

Make it a point to use ingredients that you already have on hand whenever possible. Alternatively, make sure that all of the meals that you eat during the week use very similar ingredients. When you do this, you know that you're avoiding causing any waste or losing ingredients along the way, meaning that you can save money. The good news is, on the Mediterranean diet, there are plenty of delicious meals that enjoy very similar ingredients that you can eat.

Avoid Recipes that Call for a Special Ingredient

If you're trying to avoid waste, it is a good idea for you to avoid any ingredients in meals that are not going to carry over to other meals during your weekly plan. By avoiding doing so, you can usually save yourself that money for that one ingredient that would be wasted. Alternatively, if you find that you really want that dish, try seeing if you can freeze some of it for later. When you do that, you can usually ensure that your special ingredient at least didn't go to waste.

Use Seasonal Foods

Fruits and veggies are usually cheaper when you buy them in season, and even better, when you do so, you will be enjoying a basic factor of the Mediterranean diet just by virtue of enjoying the foods when they are fresh. Fresher foods are usually tastier, and they also tend to carry more vitamins and minerals because they have not had the chance to degrade over time.

Make Use of Leftovers and Extra Portions

One of the greatest things that you can do when it comes to meal planning is to make use of your leftovers and make-ahead meals. When you do this regularly, making larger portions than you need, you can then use the extras as lunches and dinners all week long, meaning that you won't have to be constantly worrying about the food that you eat for lunch. We will use some of these in the meal plans that you will see as well.

Eat What You Enjoy

Finally, the last thing to remember with your meal plan is that you ought to be enjoying the foods that are on it at all times. When you ensure that the foods that you have on your plate are those that you actually enjoy, sticking to your meal plan doesn't become such a chore, and that means that you will be able to do better as well with your own diet. Your meal plan should be loaded up with foods that you are actually excited about enjoying. Meal planning and dieting should not be a drag—you should love every moment of it!

Chapter 2: 1 Month Meal Plan

This meal plan is designed to be used for one month to help you simplify making sure that you have delicious meals to eat without having to think. These meals are fantastic options if you don't know where to start but want to enjoy your Mediterranean diet without much hassle. For each of the five weeks included, you will get one breakfast recipe, one lunch recipe, one dinner recipe, and one snack recipe to make meal planning a breeze. So, give these recipes a try! Many of them are so delicious, you'll want to enjoy them over and over again!

Week 1: Success is no accident—you have to reach for it

Mediterranean Breakfast Sandwich

Serves: 4

Time: 20 minutes

Ingredients:

- Baby spinach (2 c.)

- Eggs (4)

- Fresh rosemary (1 Tbsp.)

- Low-fat feta cheese (4 Tbsp.)

- Multigrain sandwich thins (4)

- Olive oil (4 tsp.)

- Salt and pepper according to preference

- Tomato (1, cut into 8 slices)

Instructions:

1. Preheat your oven. This recipe works best at 375° F. Cut the sandwich things in half and brush the insides with half of your olive oil. Place the things on a baking sheet and toast for about five minutes or until the edges are lightly browned and crispy.

2. In a large skillet, heat the rest of your olive oil and the rosemary. Use medium-high heat. Crack your eggs into the skillet one at a time. Cook until the whites have set while keeping the yolks runny. Break the yolks and flip the eggs until done.

3. Serve by placing spinach in between two sandwich thins, along with two tomato slices, an egg, and a tablespoon of feta cheese.

Greek Chicken Bowls

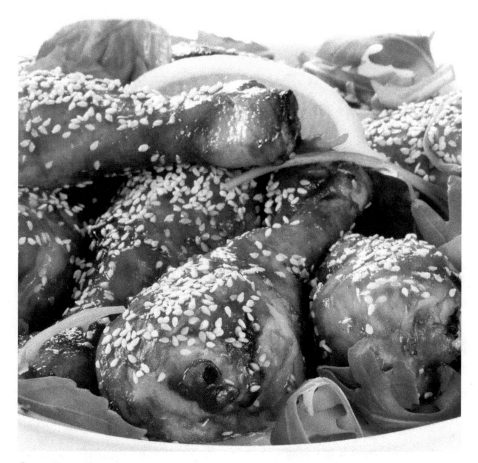

Serves: 4

Time: 20 minutes

Ingredients:

- Arugula (4 c.)
- Chicken breast tenders (1 lb.)

- Cucumber (1, diced)
- Curry powder (1 Tbsp.)
- Dried basil (1 tsp.)
- Garlic powder (1 tsp.)
- Kalamata olives (2 Tbsp.)
- Olive oil (1 Tbsp.)
- Pistachios (0.25 c., chopped)
- Red onion (half, sliced)
- Sunflower seeds (0.25 c.)
- Tzatziki sauce (1 c.)

Instructions:

1. In a bowl, mix in the chicken tenders, curry powder, dried basil, and garlic powder. Make sure to coat the chicken evenly.
2. Heat one tablespoon of olive oil over medium-high. Add the chicken and cook for about four minutes on each side. Remove from the pan and set aside to cool.
3. Place one cup of arugula into four bowls. Toss in the diced cucumber, onion, and kalamata olives.
4. Chop the chicken and distribute evenly between the four bowls.
5. Top with tzatziki sauce, pistachio seeds, and sunflower seeds.

Ratatouille

Serves: 8

Time: 1 hour 30 minutes

Ingredients:

- Crushed tomatoes (1 28 oz. can)
- Eggplants (2)
- Fresh basil (4 Tbsp., chopped)
- Fresh parsley (2 Tbsp., chopped)
- Fresh thyme (2 tsp.)
- Garlic cloves (4, minced and 1 tsp, minced)
- Olive oil (6 Tbsp.)
- Onion (1, diced)
- Red bell pepper (1, diced)
- Roma tomatoes (6)
- Salt and pepper to personal preference
- Yellow bell pepper (1, diced)
- Yellow squashes (2)
- Zucchinis (2)

Instructions:

1. Get your oven ready. This recipe works best at 375° F.
2. Slice the tomatoes, eggplant, squash, and zucchini into thin rounds and set them to the side.

3. Heat up two tablespoons of olive oil in an oven safe pan using medium-high heat. Sauté your onions, four cloves of garlic, and bell peppers for about ten minutes or when soft. Add in your pepper and salt along with the full can of crushed tomatoes. Add in two tablespoons of basil. Stir thoroughly.

4. Take the vegetable slices from earlier and arrange them on top of the sauce in a pattern of your choosing. For example, a slice of eggplant, followed by a slice of tomato, squash, and zucchini, then repeating. Start from the outside and work inward to the center of your pan. Sprinkle salt and pepper overtop the veggies.

5. In a bowl, toss in the remaining basil and garlic, thyme, parsley, salt, pepper, and the rest of the olive oil. Mix it all together, and spoon over the veggies.

6. Cover your pan and bake for 40 minutes. Uncover and then continue baking for another 20 minutes.

Snack Platter

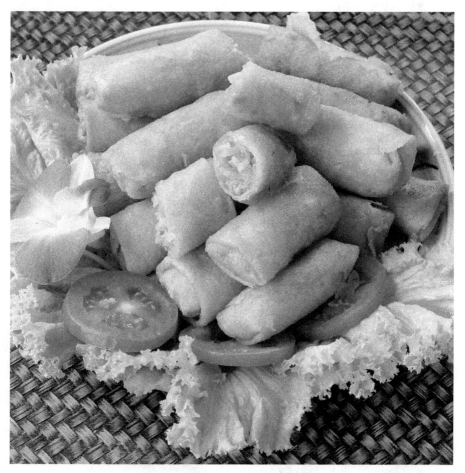

Serves: 6

Time:

Ingredients:

Rosemary Almonds

- Butter (1 Tbsp.)

- Dried rosemary (2 tsp.)
- Salt (pinch)
- Whole almonds (2 c.)

Hummus

- Chickpeas (1 15 oz. can, drained and rinsed)
- Garlic clove (1, peeled)
- Lemon (half, juiced)
- Olive oil (2 Tbsp.)
- Salt and pepper according to personal preference
- Tahini (2 Tbsp.)
- Water (2 Tbsp.)

Other sides

- Bell pepper (1, sliced)
- Cucumber (1, sliced)
- Feta cheese (4 oz, cubed)
- Kalamata olives (handful, drained)
- Pepperoncini peppers (6, drained)
- Pitas (6, sliced into wedges)
- Small fresh mozzarella balls (18)
- Soppressata (6 oz.)
- Sweet cherry peppers (18)

Instructions:

1. To get started, make your rosemary almonds. Take a large skillet and place it on a burner set to medium heat. Start melting the butter in, then toss in the almonds, rosemary and a bit of salt. Toss the nuts on occasion to ensure even coating.

2. Cook the almonds for roughly ten minutes, getting them nicely toasted. Set the almonds off to the side to let them cool.

3. Now you'll set out to make the hummus. Take a blender or food processor and toss in the hummus ingredients. Blend until you get a nice, smooth paste. If you find that your paste is too thick, try blending in a bit of water until you get the desired consistency. Once you have the right consistency, taste for seasoning and adjust as necessary.

4. Pour and scrape the hummus into a bowl and drizzle in a bit of olive oil. Set it off to the side to get the rest of the platter going.

5. Grab the sweet cherry peppers and stuff them with the little balls of mozzarella. Arrange a platter in any pattern you like. If serving for a party or family, try keeping each snack in its own little segment to keep things looking neat.

Week 2: Self-belief and effort will take you to what you want to achieve

Breakfast Quesadilla

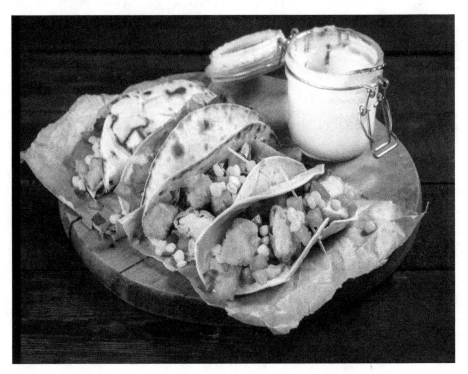

Serves: 1

Time: 10 minutes

Ingredients:

- Basil (handful)
- Eggs (2)
- Flour tortilla (1)

- Green pesto (1 tsp.)
- Mozzarella (0.25 c.)
- Salt and pepper according to personal preference
- Tomato (half, sliced)

Instructions:

1. Scramble your eggs until just a little runny. Remember, you will be cooking them further inside the quesadilla. Season with salt and pepper.
2. Take the eggs and spread over half of the tortilla.
3. Add basil, pesto, mozzarella cheese, and the slices of tomato.
4. Fold your tortilla and toast on an oiled pan. Toast until both sides are golden brown.

Greek Orzo Salad

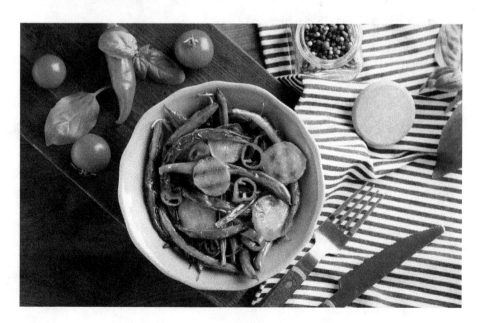

Serves: 6

Time: 25 minutes

Ingredients:

- Canned chickpeas (1 c., drained and rinsed)
- Dijon mustard (0.5 tsp)
- Dill (0.33 c., chopped)
- Dried oregano (1 tsp)
- English cucumber (half, diced)
- Feta cheese crumbles (0.5 c.)
- Kalamata olives (0.33 c., halved)
- Lemon (half, juice and zest)
- Mint (0.33 c., chopped)
- Olive oil (3 Tbsp.)
- Orzo pasta (1.25 c. when dry)
- Roasted red pepper (half, diced)
- Salt and pepper to taste
- Shallot (0.25 c., minced)
- White wine vinegar (2 Tbsp.)

Instructions:

1. Prepare the orzo according to the packaging details. Once the orzo is al dente, drain it and rinse until it drops to room temperature.

2. In a bowl, toss all the ingredients together until thoroughly incorporated.

One Pot Mediterranean Chicken

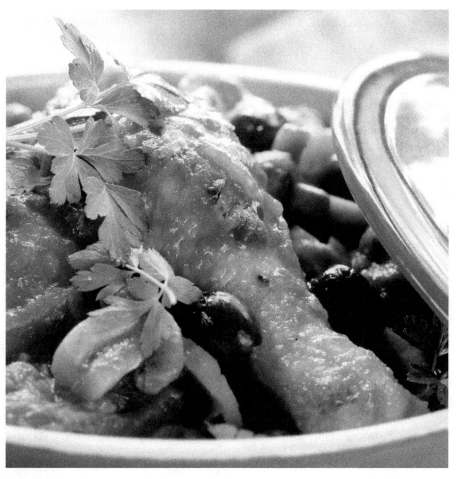

Serves: 4

Time: 1 hour

Ingredients:

- Chicken broth (3 c.)
- Chicken thighs (3, bone in, skin on)
- Chickpeas (1 15 oz can, drained and rinsed)
- Dried oregano (0.5 tsp.)
- Fresh parsley (2 Tbsp., chopped)
- Garlic cloves (2, minced)
- Kalamata olives (0.75 c., halved)
- Olive oil (2 tsp.)
- Onion (1, finely diced)
- Orzo pasta (8 ounces uncooked)
- Roasted peppers (0.5 c., chopped)
- Salt and pepper according to personal preference

Instructions:

1. Prepare your oven at 375°. Heat your olive oil in a large skillet over medium-high heat.
2. Season the chicken with salt and pepper on both sides. Toss the chicken into the skillet and cook for five minutes on each side, or until golden in color. Remove the chicken.
3. Take the skillet and drain most of the rendered fat, leaving about a teaspoon. Add the onion and cook for five minutes. Toss in the garlic and cook for an additional minute.
4. Now you will want to add the orzo, roasted peppers, oregano, chickpeas, and olives into the pan. Add in salt and pepper.
5. Place the thighs on top of the orzo and pour in the chicken broth.
6. Bring to a boil, then cover and place in the oven. Bake for 35 minutes or until chicken has cooked through. Top with parsley and serve.

Mediterranean Nachos

Serves: 6

Time: 10 minutes

Ingredients:

- Canned artichoke hearts (1 c., rinsed, drained, and dried)
- Canned garbanzo beans (0.75 c., rinsed, drained, and dried)
- Feta cheese (0.5 c., crumbled)
- Fresh cilantro (2 Tbsp., chopped)
- Pine nuts (2.5 Tbsp.)
- Roasted red peppers (0.5 c., dried)
- Sabra Hummus (half of their 10 oz. container)
- Tomatoes (0.5 c., chopped)
- Tortilla chips (roughly half a bag)

Instructions:

1. Get your oven ready by setting it to 375°F. In a baking pan, layer the tortilla chips, and spread hummus over them evenly. Top with garbanzo beans, red peppers, artichoke hearts, feta cheese, and pine nuts.

2. Bake for about five minutes or until warmed through. Remove the baking pan and top the nachos with fresh cilantro and tomatoes. Serve and enjoy.

Week 3: The harder you work, the greater the success

Breakfast Tostadas

Serves: 4

Time: 15 minutes

Ingredients:

- Beaten eggs (8)
- Cucumber (0.5 c., seeded and chopped)
- Feta (0.25 c., crumbled)
- Garlic powder (0.5 tsp)
- Green onions (0.5 c., chopped)
- Oregano (0.5 tsp)
- Red Pepper (0.5 c., diced)
- Roasted red pepper hummus (0.5 c.)
- Skim milk (0.5 c.)
- Tomatoes (0.5 c., diced)
- Tostadas (4)

Instructions:

1. In a large skillet, cook the red pepper for two minutes on medium heat until softened. Toss in the eggs, garlic powder, milk, oregano, and green onions. Stir constantly until the egg whites have set.
2. Top the tostadas with hummus, egg mixture, cucumber, feta, and tomatoes.

Roasted Vegetable Bowl

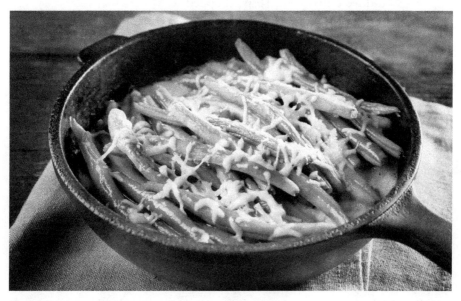

Serves: 2

Time: 45 minutes

Ingredients:

- Crushed red pepper flakes (a pinch)
- Fresh parsley (1 Tbsp., chopped)
- Kalamata olives (0.25 c.)

- Kale (1 c., ribboned)

- Lemon juice (1 Tbsp.)

- Marinated artichoke hearts (0.25 c., drained and chopped)

- Nutritional yeast (1 Tbsp.)

- Olive oil (1 Tbsp., then enough to drizzle)

- Salt and pepper to taste

- Spaghetti squash (half, seeds removed)

- Sun-dried tomatoes (2 Tbsp., chopped)

- Walnuts (0.25 c., chopped)

Instructions:

1. Get your oven ready by setting it to 400° F. Take a baking sheet and blanket it with parchment paper.
2. Take the squash half and place it on the parchment paper. Drizzle olive oil over the side that is cut, and season with salt and pepper. Turn it over so it is facing cut side down and bake for 40 minutes. It is ready when it is soft.
3. Remove the squash shell, and season with a bit more salt and pepper.
4. Stack the kale, artichoke hearts, walnuts, sun-dried tomatoes, and kalamata olives on the squash.
5. Squeeze the lemon juice over and drizzle olive oil. Finish with chopped parsley and a bit of crushed red pepper flakes.

Mediterranean Chicken

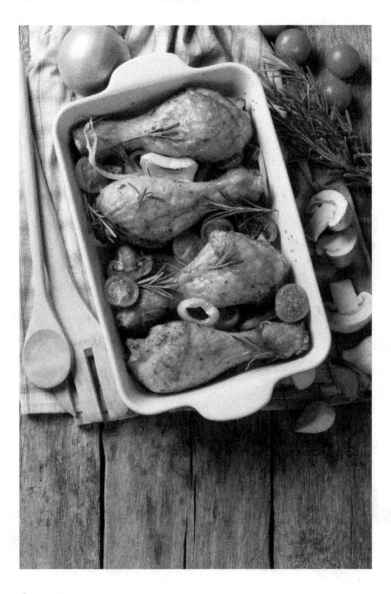

Serves: 4

Time: 40 minutes

Ingredients:

- Chicken breasts (1 lb., boneless, skinless)
- Chives (2 Tbsp., chopped)
- Feta cheese (0.25 c., crumbled)
- Garlic (1 tsp., minced)
- Italian seasoning (1 tsp.)
- Lemon juice (2 Tbsp.)
- Olive oil (2 Tbsp., and 1 Tbsp.)
- Salt and pepper according to personal preference
- Tomatoes (1 c., diced)

Instructions:

1. Pour in two tablespoons of olive oil, the lemon juice, salt, pepper, garlic, and Italian seasoning in a resealable plastic bag. Add in the chicken, seal and shake to coat the chicken.
2. Allow the chicken to marinate for at least 30 minutes in the refrigerator.
3. Heat the rest of the olive oil in a pan over medium heat.
4. Place the chicken on the pan and cook for five minutes on each side, or until cooked through.
5. In a bowl, mix the tomatoes, chives, and feta cheese. Season with salt and pepper.
6. When serving, spoon the tomato mixture on top of the chicken.

Baked Phyllo Chips

Serves: 2

Time: 10 minutes

Ingredients:

- Grated cheese (your choice)
- Olive oil (enough to brush with)
- Phyllo sheets (4)
- Salt and pepper according to personal preference

Instructions:

1. Get your oven ready by setting it to 350° F. Brush olive oil over a phyllo sheet generously. Sprinkle grated cheese and your seasoning on top.
2. Grab a second sheet of your phyllo and place it on top of the first one. Again, brush with olive oil and sprinkle cheese and seasoning on top.
3. Repeat this process with the remaining sheets of phyllo. Top the stack with cheese and seasoning.
4. Once complete, cut the stack of phyllo into bite-sized rectangles. A pizza cutter may be helpful here.
5. Grab a baking sheet and blanket it with some parchment paper. Take your phyllo rectangles and place them on the parchment paper.
6. Bake in the oven for about seven minutes or until they reach a golden color.
7. Remove them from the oven and allow them to cool before serving.

Week 4: You don't need perfection—you need effort

Mini Omelets

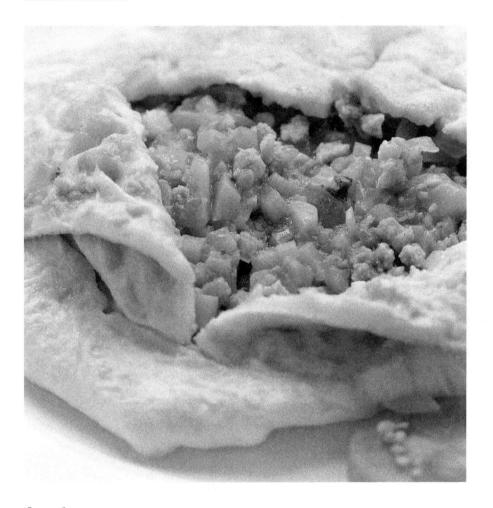

Serves: 8

Time: 40 minutes

Ingredients:

- Cheddar cheese (0.25 c., shredded)
- Eggs (8)
- Half and half (0.5 c.)
- Olive oil (2 tsps.)
- Salt and pepper according to personal preference
- Spinach (1 c., chopped)

Instructions:

1. Get your oven ready by setting it to 350° F. Prepare a muffin pan or ramekins by greasing them with olive oil.
2. In a bowl, beat the eggs and dairy until you have a fluffy consistency.
3. Stir in the cheese and your seasonings. Pour in the spinach and continue beating the eggs.
4. Pour the egg mixture into your ramekins or muffin pan.
5. Bake the omelets until they have set, which should be roughly 25 minutes. Remove them from the oven and allow them to cool before serving.

Basil Shrimp Salad

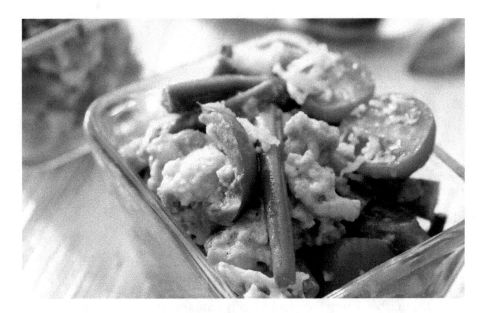

Serves: 2

Time: 40 minutes

Ingredients:

- Dried basil (1 tsp.)
- Lemon juice (1 Tbsp.)
- Olive oil (1 tsp.)
- Romaine lettuce (2 c.)
- Shrimp (12 medium or 8 large)
- White wine vinegar (0.25 c.)

Instructions:

1. Whisk together the white wine vinegar, olive oil, lemon juice, and basil. Stick your shrimp in the marinade for half an hour.
2. Take the marinade and shrimp and cook in a skillet over medium heat until cooked through.
3. Allow the shrimp to cool along with the juice and pour into a bowl. Toss in the romaine lettuce and mix well to get the flavor thoroughly infused in the salad. Serve.

Mediterranean Flounder

Serves: 4

Time: 40 minutes

Ingredients:

- Capers (0.25 c.)
- Diced tomatoes (1 can)
- Flounder fillets (1 lb.)
- Fresh basil (12 leaves, chopped)
- Fresh parmesan cheese (3 Tbsp., grated)
- Garlic cloves (2, chopped)
- Italian seasoning (a pinch)
- Kalamata olives (0.5 c., pitted and chopped)
- Lemon juice (1 tsp.)

- Red onion (half, chopped)
- White wine (0.25 c.)

Instructions:

1. Set your oven to 425° F. Take a skillet and pour in enough olive oil to sauté the onion until soft. Cook on medium-high heat.
2. Toss in the garlic, Italian seasoning, and tomatoes. Cook for an additional five minutes.
3. Pour in the wine, capers, olives, lemon juice, and only half of the basil you chopped.
4. Reduce the heat to low and stir in the parmesan cheese. Simmer for ten minutes or until the sauce has thickened.
5. Place the flounder fillets in a baking pan and pour the sauce over top. Sprinkle the remaining basil on top and bake for 12 minutes.

Nutty Energy Bites

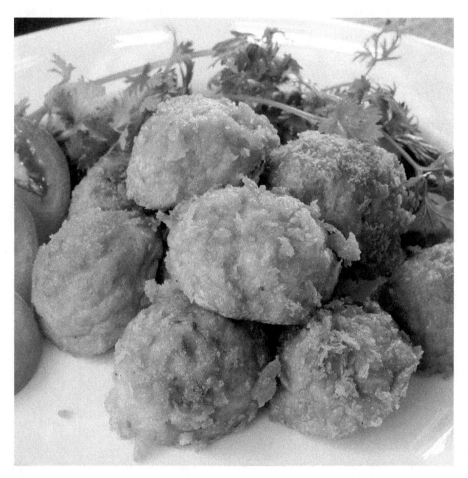

Serves: 10

Time: 10 minutes

Ingredients:

- Dried dates (1 c., pitted)
- Almonds (0.5 c.)

- Pine nuts (0.25 c.)
- Flaxseeds (1 Tbsp., milled) Porridge oats (2 Tbsp.)
- Pistachios (0.25 c., coarsely ground)

Instructions:

1. Take the dates, pine nuts, milled flaxseeds, almonds, and porridge oats and pour them into a food processor or blender. Mix until thoroughly incorporated.
2. Using a tablespoon, scoop the mixture and roll it between your hands until you have a small, bite-sized ball. Do this until you have used the entirety of the dough. This recipe should be enough for about ten.
3. On a plate, sprinkle your ground pistachios. Take the energy balls and roll them on the pistachio grounds, making sure to coat them evenly. Serve or store in the refrigerator.

Week 5: Transformation Happens One Day at a Time

Mediterranean Breakfast Bowl

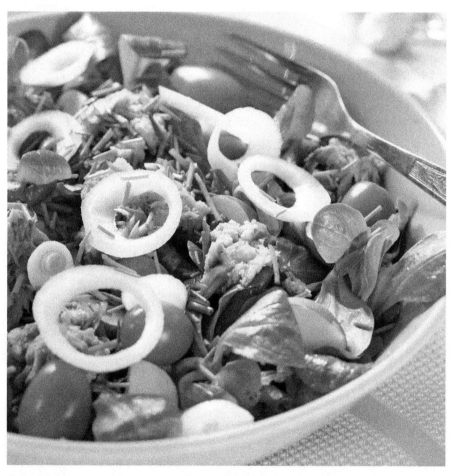

Serves: 1

Time: 25 minutes

Ingredients:

- Artichoke hearts (0.25 c., chopped)
- Baby arugula (2 c.)
- Capers (1 Tbsp.)
- Egg (1)
- Feta (2 Tbsp., crumbled)
- Garlic (0.25 tsp)
- Kalamata olives (5, chopped)
- Lemon thyme (1 Tbsp., chopped)
- Olive oil (0.5 Tbsp.)
- Pepper (0.25 tsp)
- Sun-dried tomatoes (2 Tbsp., chopped)
- Sweet potato (1 c., cubed)

Instructions:

1. Take your olive oil and, when hot, pan fry your sweet potatoes for 5-10 minutes until they have softened. Then, sprinkle on the seasonings.
2. Place arugula into a bowl, then top with potatoes, then everything but the egg.
3. Prepare the egg to your liking and serve.

Chicken Shawarma Pita Pockets

Serves: 6

Time: 40 minutes

Ingredients:

- Cayenne (0.5 tsp)
- Chicken thighs (8, boneless, skinless, bite-sized pieces)
- Cloves (0.5 tsp, ground)
- Garlic powder (0.75 Tbsp.)
- Ground cumin (0.75 Tbsp.)
- Lemon juice (1 lemon)
- Olive oil (0.33 c.)
- Onion (1, sliced thinly)
- Paprika (0.75 Tbsp.)
- Salt
- Turmeric powder (0.75 Tbsp.)

To serve:

- Pita pockets (6)
- Tzatziki sauce
- Arugula
- Diced tomatoes
- Diced onions
- Sliced Kalamata olives

Instructions:

1. Combine all spices. Then, place all chicken, already diced, into the bowl. Coat well, then toss in onions, lemon juice, and oil. Mix well and let marinade for at least 3 hours, or overnight.

2. Preheat the oven to 425 F. Allow chicken to sit at room temperature a few minutes. Then, spread it on an oiled sheet pan. Roast for 30 minutes.

3. To serve, fill up a pita pocket with tzatziki, chicken, arugula, and any toppings you prefer. Enjoy.

Turkey Mediterranean Casserole

Serves: 6

Time: 35 minutes

Ingredients:

- Fusilli pasta (0.5 lbs.)
- Turkey (1.5 c., chopped)
- Sun dried tomatoes (2 Tbsp., drained)
- Canned artichokes (7 oz., drained)
- Kalamata olives (3.5 oz., drained and chopped)
- Parsley (0.5 Tbsp., chopped and fresh)
- Basil (1 T, fresh)
- Salt and pepper to taste

- Marinara sauce (1 c.)
- Black chopped olives (2 oz., drained)
- Mozzarella cheese (1.5 c., shredded)

Instructions:

1. Warm your oven to 350 F. Prepare your pasta according to the directions, drain, and place into a bowl. Prepare your basil, parsley, olives, tomatoes, artichokes, and other ingredients.
2. Mix together the pasta with the turkey, tomatoes, olives, artichokes, herbs, seasoning, and marinara sauce. Give it a good mix to incorporate all of the ingredients evenly.
3. Take a 9x13 oven-safe dish and layer in the first half of your pasta mixture. Then, sprinkle on half of your mozzarella cheese. Top with the rest of the pasta, then sprinkle on the chopped black olives as well. Spread the rest of the shredded cheese on top, then bake it for 20-25 minutes. It is done when the cheese is all bubbly and the casserole is hot.

Heirloom Tomato and Cucumber Toast

Serves: 2

Time: 5 minutes

Ingredients:

- Heirloom tomato (1, diced)
- Persian cucumber (1, diced)
- Extra virgin olive oil (1 tsp)
- Oregano (a pinch, dried)
- Kosher salt and pepper
- Whipped cream cheese (2 tsp)
- Whole grain bread (2 pieces)
- Balsamic glaze (1 tsp)

Instructions:

4. Combine the tomato, cucumber, oil, and all seasonings together.
5. Spread cheese across bread, then top with mixture, followed by balsamic glaze.

Chapter 3: Maintaining Your Diet

Sticking to a diet can be tough. You could see that other people are having some great food and wish that you could enjoy it too. You might realize that you miss the foods that you used to eat and feel like it's a drag to not be able to enjoy them. When you are able to enjoy the foods that you are eating, sticking to your diet is far easier. However, that doesn't mean that you won't miss those old foods sometimes. Thankfully, the Mediterranean diet is not a very restrictive one—you are able to enjoy foods in moderation that would otherwise not be allowed, and because of that, you can take the slice of cake at the work party, or you can choose to pick up a coffee for yourself every now and then. When you do this, you're not doing anything wrong, so long as you enjoy food in moderation.

Within this chapter, we are going to take a look at several tips that you can use that will help you with maintaining your diet so that you will be able to stick to it, even when you feel like things are getting difficult. Think of this as your guide to avoiding giving in entirely—this will help you to do the best thing for yourself so that you can know that you are healthy. Now, let's get started.

Find Your Motivation

First, if you want to keep yourself on your diet, one of the best things that you can do is make sure that you find and stick to your motivation. Make sure that you know what it is in life that is motivating you. Are you losing weight because a doctor told you to? Fair enough—but how do you make that personal and about yourself? Maybe instead of looking at it as a purely health-related choice, look at it as something that you are doing because of yourself. Maybe you are eating better so that you are able to watch your children graduate or so that you can run after them at the park and stay healthy, even when it is hard to do so.

Remind Yourself Why You are Eating Healthily

When you find that you are struggling to eat healthily, remind yourself of why you are doing it in the first place. When you do this enough, you will begin to resist the urges easier than ever. Make it a point to tell yourself not to eat something a certain way. Take the time to remind yourself that you don't need to order that greasy pizza—you are eating better foods because you want to be there for your children or grandchildren.

Reminding yourself of your motivation is a great way to overcome those cravings that you may have at any point in time. The cravings that you have are usually strong and compelling, but if you learn to overcome them, you realize that they weren't actually as powerful as you thought they were. Defeat the cravings. Learn to tell yourself that they are not actually able to control you. Tell yourself that you can do better with yourself.

Eat Slowly

Now, on the Mediterranean diet, you should already be eating your meals with other people anyway. You should be taking the time to enjoy those meals while talking to other people and ensuring that you get that connection with them, and in doing so, you realize that you are able to do better. You realize that you are able to keep yourself under control longer, and that is a great way to defend and protect yourself from overeating.

When you eat slowly, you can get the same effect. Eating slowly means that you will have longer for your brain to realize that you should be eating less. When you are able to trigger that sensation of satiety because you were eating slowly, you end up eating fewer calories by default, and that matters immensely.

Keep Yourself Accountable

Don't forget that, ultimately, your diet is something that you must control on your own. Keep yourself accountable by making sure that you show other people what you are doing. If you are trying to lose weight, let them know, and tell them how you plan to do so. When you do this, you are able to remind yourself that other people know what you are doing and why—this is a great way to foster that sense of accountability because you will feel like you have to actually follow through, or you will be embarrassed by having to admit fault. You could also make accountability to yourself as well. When you do this, you are able to remind yourself that your diet is your own. Using apps to track your food and caloric intake is just one way that you can do this.

Remember Your Moderation

While it can be difficult to face a diet where you feel like you can't actually enjoy the foods that you would like to eat, the truth is that on the Mediterranean diet, you are totally okay to eat those foods that you like or miss if you do so in moderation. There is nothing that is absolutely forbidden on the Mediterranean diet—there are just foods that you should be restricting regularly. However, that doesn't mean that you can't have a treat every now and then.

Remembering to live in moderation will help you from feeling like you have to cheat or give up as well. When you are able to enjoy your diet and still enjoy the times where you want to enjoy your treats, you realize that there is actually a happy medium between sticking to the diet and deciding to quit entirely.

Identify the Difference between Hunger and Craving

Another great way to help yourself stick to your diet is to recognize that there is a very real difference between actually being hungry and just craving something to eat. In general, cravings are felt in the mouth—when you feel like you are salivating or like you need to eat something, but it is entirely in your head and mouth, you know that you have a craving. When you are truly hungry, you feel an emptiness in your stomach—you are able to know because your abdomen is where the motivation is coming from.

Being able to tell when you have a craving and when you are genuinely hungry, you can usually avoid eating extra calories that you didn't actually need. This is major—if you don't want to overeat, you need to know when your body actually needs something and when it just wants something. And if you find that you just want something, that's okay too—just find a way to move on from it. If you want to indulge a bit here and there, there's no harm in that!

Stick to the Meal Plan

When it comes to sticking to a diet, one of the easiest and most straightforward ways to do so is to just stick to your meal plan that you set up. You have it there for a reason—it is there for you to fall back on, and the sooner that you are willing to accept that, recognizing that ultimately, you can stay on track when you don't have to think about things too much, the better you will do. You will be able to succeed on your diet because you will know that you have those tools in place to protect you—they will be lined up to ensure that your diet is able to provide you with everything that you need and they will also be there so that you can know that you are on the right track.

Drink Plenty of Water

Another key to keeping yourself on track with your diet is to make sure that you drink plenty of water throughout the day. Oftentimes, we mistake our thirst with hunger and eat instead. Of course, if you're thirsty, food isn't going to really fix your problem, and you will end up continuing to mix up the sensation as you try to move past it. The more you eat, the thirstier you will get until you realize that you're full but still feeling "hungry." By drinking plenty of water any time that you think that you might want to eat, you will be able to keep yourself hydrated, and in addition, you will prevent yourself from unintentionally eating too much.

Eat Several Times Per Day

One of the best ways to keep yourself on track with your diet is to make sure that you are regularly eating. By eating throughout the day, making sure that you keep yourself full, it is easier to keep yourself strong enough to resist giving in to cravings or anything else. When you do this regularly, you will discover that you can actually keep away much of your cravings so that you are more successful in managing your diet.

Eating several times per day often involves small meals and snacks if you prefer to do so. Some people don't like doing this, but if you find that you're one of those people who will do well on a diet when you are never actually hungry enough to get desperate enough to break it, you will probably be just fine.

Fill Up on Protein

Another great way to protect yourself from giving in and caving on your diet is to make sure that you fill up on protein. Whether it comes from an animal or plant source, make sure that every time you eat, you have some sort of tangible protein source. This is the best way to keep yourself on track because protein keeps you fuller for longer. When you eat something that's loaded up with protein, you don't feel the need to eat as much later on. The protein is usually very dense, and that means that you get to resist feeling hungry for longer than you thought that you would.

Some easy proteins come from nuts—but make sure that you are mindful that you do not end up overeating during this process—you might unintentionally end up eating too many without realizing it. While you should be eating proteins regularly, make sure that you are mindful of calorie content as well!

Keep Only Healthy Foods

A common mistake that people make while dieting is that they end up caving when they realize that their home is filled up with foods that they shouldn't be eating. Perhaps you are the only person in your home that is attempting to diet. In this case, you may end up running into a situation where you have all sorts of non-compliant foods on hand. You might have chips for your kids or snacks that your partner likes to eat on hand. You may feel like it is difficult for you to stay firm when you have that to consider, and that means that you end up stuck in temptation.

One of the best ways to prevent this is to either cut all of the unhealthy junk out of your home entirely or make sure that you keep the off-limits foods in specific places so that you don't have to look at it and see it tempting you every time that you go to get a snack for yourself. By trying to keep yourself limited to just healthy foods, you will be healthier, and you will make better decisions.

Eat Breakfast Daily

Finally, make sure that breakfast is non-negotiable. Make sure that you enjoy it every single day, even if you're busy. This is where those make-ahead meals can come in handy; by knowing that you have to keep to a meal plan and knowing that you already have the food on hand, you can keep yourself fed. Breakfast sets you up for success or failure—if you want to truly succeed on your diet, you must make sure that you are willing to eat those healthier foods as much as possible, and you must get started on the right foot. Enjoy those foods first thing every day. Eat so that you are not ravenous when you finally do decide that it is time to sit down and find something to eat. Even if you just have a smoothie or something quick to eat as you go, having breakfast will help you to persevere.

PART II

What Is Fasting and Why You Should Do It

Chapter 1: What Is Fasting?

Introduction to Fasting

Latest Research and Studies about Fasting

In a research published by the Springer Journal, it was found that fasting helps fight against obesity. The study, led by Kyoung Han Kim and Yun Hye Kim, was aimed at tracking the effects of fasting on fat cells. They put a group of mice into a four-month period of intermittent fasts, where the mice were fed for two days, followed by a day of fasting. In the end, the group of fasting mice was found to weigh less than the non-fasting mice, even though all of them had consumed exact quantities of food. The group of fasting mice had registered a drop in the fat buildup around fat cells. The explanation was that the fat had been converted into energy when glucose was insufficient. (www.sciencedaily.com/releases/2017/10/171017110041.htm)

In November 2017, Harvard researchers established that fasting can induce a long life, as well as minimize aging effects. It was found that fasting revitalizes mitochondria. Mitochondria are the organelles that act as body power plants. In this replenished state, mitochondria optimize physiological functions, in effect slowing down the aging process. Fasting also promotes low blood glucose levels, which improves skin clarity and boosts the immune system. (https://newatlas.com/fasting-increase-lifespan-mitochondria-harvard/52058/)

Sebastian Brandhorst, a researcher based at the University of Southern California, found out that fasting has a positive impact on brain health. Fasting induces low blood sugar levels, causing the liver to produce ketone bodies that pass on to the brain in place of sugars. Ketone bodies are much more stable and efficient energy sources than glucose.

Researchers from the same university have posited that fasting minimizes chances of coming down with diabetes and other degenerative diseases. Moreover, they discovered that fasting induces low production of the IGF-1 hormone, which is a catalyst in aging and spread of disease. (https://www.cnbc.com/2017/10/20/science-diet-fasting-may-be-more-important-than-just-eating-less.html)

Biological Effects of Fasting

- **Cleanses the body**

Our bodies harbor an endless count of toxins, and these toxins announce their presence through symptoms like low energy, infections, allergies, terrible moods, bloating, confusion, and so on.

Eliminating toxins from your body will do you a world of good in the sense that your body will upgrade and start functioning optimally. There are many ways to cleanse your body: hydrotherapy, meditation, organic diets, herbs, yoga, etc.

But one of the most effective ways of cleansing your body is through fasting. When you go on a fast, you allow the body to channel the energy that would have been used for digestion into flushing out toxins.

- **Improves heart health**

Studies show that people who undertake regular fasts are less likely to contract coronary infections. Fasting fights against obesity, and obesity is a recipe for heart disease. It purifies the blood too, in that sense augmenting the flow of blood around the body.

- **Improves the immune system**

Fasting rids the body of toxins and radicals, thus boosting the body's immune system and minimizes the chances of coming down with degenerative diseases like cancer. Fasting reduces inflammation as well.

- **Improves bowel movement**

One of the problems of consuming food on the regular is that the food sort of clogs up your stomach, causing indigestion. You might go for days without visiting the bathroom to perform number two. But when you fast, your body resources won't be bogged down by loads of undigested foods, and so your bowel movement will be seamless. Also, fasting promotes healthy gut bacteria.

- **Induces alertness**

When your stomach is full because of combined undigested foods (i.e., "garbage"), you are more likely to experience brain-fog. You won't have any concentration on the tasks at hand. You will just sit around and laze the hours away, belching and spitting. But when you fast, your mind will be clear so it will be easy to cultivate focus.

Treating Fasting as a Lifestyle Choice

When you perform a simple Google search for the word "fasting," millions of results come up. Fasting is slowly becoming a mainstream subject. This is mostly because of the research-backed evidence that has been published by many reputable publications listing down the various benefits of fasting such as improved brain health, increased production of the human growth hormone, a stronger immune system, heart health, and weight loss—thus its appeal to health-conscious people as a catalyst for their health goals.

Taking up fasting as a lifestyle choice will see you go without food for anywhere from a couple of hours to days. But before you get into it, you'd do yourself a world of good to first obtain clearance from a physician, certifying that your body is ready, because not everyone is made for it. For instance, the symptoms of illnesses such as cancer may worsen after a long stretch of food deprivation. So people with degenerative diseases such as cancer should consider getting professional help or staying away altogether. Pregnant women, malnourished people, and children are advised to stay clear too.

The first thing you must do is to establish your fasting routine. For instance, you may choose to skip breakfast, making lunch your first meal of the day. Go at it with consistency. Also, you may decide to space your meals over some hours; so that when the set hours elapse, you reach your eating window, and then go back to fasting. The real challenge is staying committed. You will find that it will be difficult to break the cycle of eating that your body had been accustomed to, but when you persevere; your body will, of course, adjust to your new habit. If you decide to go for days without food, the results will be far pronounced, but please remember to hydrate your body constantly to flush out toxins.

Summary

Fasting is the willing abstinence from food over a period of time with the goal of improving your life. Conventionally, fasting has been tied to religious practices, but a new school of thought has emerged to proclaim the health benefits of fasting—particularly, weight loss. When you go into a fast, you create a caloric deficit, which triggers the body to convert its fat stores into energy. Numerous studies by mainstream health organizations have been done on fasting, and researchers have established that fasting has a host of advantages like improved motor skills, cognition, and moods. Some of the biological effects of fasting include improved bowel movement, immune system, and heart health. If you are starting out with fasting, you must create a routine and abide by it. Not everyone is fit to practice fasting. Some of the people advised to stay away from the practice include extremely sick people, pregnant women, the malnourished, and children. If you undertake a prolonged fast, you should hydrate your body constantly.

Chapter 2: Obesity and the Standard American Diet

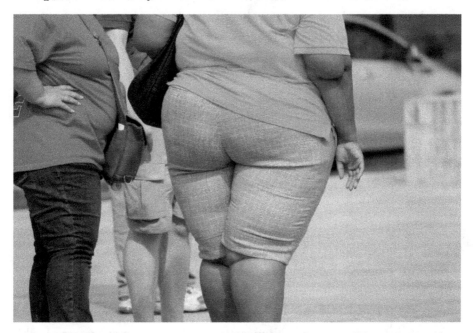

The Obesity Epidemic

We are killing ourselves with nothing more than a spoon and a fork. In 2017, obesity claimed more lives than car accidents, terrorism, and Alzheimer's combined. And the numbers are climbing at a jaw-dropping rate. Obesity has become a crisis that we cannot afford to ignore anymore.

You'd be mistaken to think that obesity is a crisis in first-world economies alone. Even developing nations are experiencing an upsurge of obese citizens. Here comes the big question: what is the **main** force behind this epidemic?

According to new research published in the New England Journal of Medicine, excessive caloric intake and lack of exercise are to blame.

Most American fast food chains have now become global. Fast foods, which are particularly calorie-laden, appeal to a lot of people across the world because of their low prices and taste. So, most people get hooked on the fast food diet and slowly begin the plunge into obesity.

The United States recognizes obesity as a health crisis and lawmakers have petitioned for tax increment on fast foods and sugary drinks, except that for a person who's addicted to fast foods, it would take a lot more than a price increase to discourage their food addiction. It would take a total lifestyle change.

Exercising alone won't help you; no matter how powerful your reps may be, or leg lifts or anything else you try in the gym, nothing can save you from a terrible diet.

And here's the complete shocker; the rate of childhood obesity has surpassed adulthood obesity; a terrible, terrible situation considering that childhood obesity almost always leads to heart complications in adult life.

Why Are We So Fat?

- **Poor food choices**

The number one reason why we are so fat is our poor choice of food. We eat too much of the wrong food, and most of it is not expended, so it becomes stored up as fat.

- **Bad genetics**

It's true that some people are genetically predisposed to gain more weight. Their genetics have wired them to convey abnormal hunger signals, so their bodies pressure them into consuming much more food.

- **Lack of strenuous activities**

Our modern-day lives involve only light physical tasks. Contrast that with the era of the dawn of humanity. Back then people would use up a lot of energy to perform physical activities and survive in unforgiving habitats. Most of the food they consumed would be actually utilized. But today, thanks to our technological advancement, we have been spared from taking part in laborious activities. This makes it hard to use up the energy from food, and the body opts to store it as fat.

- **Psychological issues**

Some of us react to bad moods by indulging in food—in particular, high-calorie fast foods—because the taste of fast foods appeals to our unstable emotions. When we fall in the habit of rewarding our bad moods or depression with binge eating, we unsuspectingly fall into the trap of food addiction, to the point of getting depressed when we fail to binge eat, kicking off our journey into obesity.

- **The endocrine system**

The thyroid's hormones play a critical role in the metabolic rate of a person. Ideally, a strong endocrine system means a high metabolic rate. And so, individuals who have a weakened endocrine system are much more likely to develop obesity.

The Problem with Calories

Calories are the basic units for quantifying the energy in the food we consume. A healthy man needs a daily dose of around 2500 calories to function optimally, and a woman needs 2000 calories.

This caloric target should be met through the consumption of various foods containing minerals, vitamins, antioxidants, fiber, and other important elements, and this is not hard at all to achieve if you adhere to the old-fashioned "traditional diet."

But the challenge is that nowadays, we have many foods with a high caloric count, and yet they hardly fill us up! For instance, fries, milkshake, and a burger make up nearly 2000 calories! You can see how easy it'd be to surpass the caloric limit by indulging in fast food.

When we consume more calories than we burn, our bodies store up the excess calories as fat, and as this process repeats itself over time, the fat has a compounding effect that leads to weight gain.

The only way to make your weight stable is through balancing out the energy you consume with the energy you expend. But for someone who suffers from obesity, if they'd like to have a normal weight, they must create a caloric deficit, and fasting is the surefire practice of creating such a deficit.

Besides checking your caloric intake, you might also consider improving your endocrine system and the efficiency of both your kidney and liver, because they have a direct impact on how the body burns calories. When you buy food products, always find out their caloric count to assess how well they'll fit within your daily caloric needs.

The American Diet

In a 2016 lifestyle survey, most Americans admitted that it is not easy to keep their diet clean and healthy. This isn't surprising, especially when you consider the fact that the average American consumes more than 20 pounds of sweeteners each year. The over-emphasis of sugar and fat in the American diet is the leading cause of obesity in Americans. Illnesses triggered by obesity long started marching into our homes. What we have now is a crisis. But let's find out the exact types of foods that Americans like to feast on (we are big on consuming, it's no secret).

As a melting point of cultures drawn from various parts of the world, it's kind of difficult to say exactly what the all-American favorite foods are. But the United States Department of Agriculture might shine some light on this. It listed down desserts, bread, chicken, soda, and alcohol, as the top five sources of calories among Americans. As you can see, the sugar intake is impossibly high. Interestingly, the US Department of Agriculture also noted that Americans aren't big on fruits.

Pizza may qualify as the all-time favorite snack of America, followed closely by burgers and other fast food. There is a reason why most fast food restaurants are successful in America and throughout the world.

It has also been established that the average American drinks about a gallon of soda every week. Even drinks that are supposed to have a low-calorie count end up being calorie-bombs because of the doctoring that takes place. For instance, black coffee is low on calorie, but not so if it has milk and ice cream and sugar all over it.

Summary

The first-world economies are not alone in facing the crisis of obesity. It has emerged that people in poor countries are battling obesity too. Obesity-related deaths are on the rise. In 2017, the figures were especially shocking, for they'd surpassed the death count of terrorist attacks, accidents, and Alzheimer's combined. One of the corrective measures that the US government is considering to undertake is tax increment on sugars. The chief reason why we are so fat is our poor diets. Our foods are laden with sugars and fats, and it doesn't help that our lifestyles allow us to expend only a small amount of energy, which leads to fat accumulation and consequent weight gain. The average man requires around 2500 calories for his body to act optimally whereas the average woman requires 2000 calories. The top five daily sources of calories for Americans include desserts, bread, chicken, soda, and alcohol.

Chapter 3: Benefits of Fasting

Improved Insulin Sensitivity

Insulin sensitivity refers to how positively or negatively your body cells respond to insulin. If you have a high insulin sensitivity, you will need less amount of insulin to convert the sugars in your blood into energy, whereas someone with low insulin sensitivity would need a significantly larger amount of insulin.

Low insulin sensitivity is characterized by increased blood sugar levels. In other words, the insulin produced by the body is underutilized when converting sugars into energy. Low insulin sensitivity may make you vulnerable to ailments such as cancer, heart disease, type 2 diabetes, stroke, and dementia.

Ailments and bad moods are the general causes of low insulin sensitivity. However, high insulin sensitivity is restored once the ailments and bad moods are over.

Fasting is shown to have a positive effect on insulin sensitivity, enhancing your body to use small amounts of insulin to convert blood sugar into energy.

Improved insulin sensitivity has a great impact on health: leveling up physiological functions and fighting off common symptoms of ailments like lightheadedness and lethargy.

To increase insulin sensitivity, here are some of the best practices: perform physical activities, lose weight, consume foods that are high in fiber and low in Glycemic load, improve your moods and alleviate depressed feelings, and finally, make sure to improve the quality of your sleep.

The rate of insulin sensitivity is also heavily dependent on lifestyle changes. For instance, if you take up sports and exercise, insulin sensitivity goes up, but if you become lazy and inactive, it goes down.

- **Increased Leptin Sensitivity**

Leptin is the hormone that determines whether you're experiencing hunger or full. This hormone plays a critical role in weight loss and health management, and if your body grows insensitive to it, you become susceptible to some ailments. Understanding the role of leptin in your body is critical as it goes into helping you improve your health regimen.

Whenever this hormone is secreted by the fat cells, the brain takes notice, and it tries to determine whether you are in need of food or are actually full. Leptin needs to work as normally as possible else you will receive an inaccurate signal that will cause you to either overfeed or starve yourself.

Low leptin sensitivity induces obesity. This condition is normally witnessed in people with high levels of insulin. The excessive sugars in blood are carried off by insulin into fat cells, but when there is an insulin overload, a communication crash is triggered between fat cells and the brain. This condition induces low leptin sensitivity. When this happens, your brain is unable to tell the exact amount of leptin in your blood, and as such it misleads you. Low leptin sensitivity causes the brain to continue sending out the hunger signal even after you are full. This causes you to eat more than you should and, given time, leads to chronic weight gain.

Fasting has been shown to increase leptin sensitivity, a state that allows the brain to be precise in determining blood leptin quantities, and ensures that the accurate signal is transmitted to control your eating habits.

- **Normalized Ghrelin Levels**

Known as the "hunger hormone," ghrelin is instrumental in regulating both appetite and the rate of energy distribution into body cells.

Increased levels of ghrelin cause the brain to trigger hunger pangs and secrete gastric acids as the body anticipates you to consume food.

It is also important to note that both ghrelin and leptin receptors are located on the same group of brain cells, even though these hormones play contrasting roles, i.e., ghrelin being the hunger hormone, and leptin the satiety hormone.

The primary role of ghrelin is to increase appetite and see to it that the body has a larger fat reservoir. So, high ghrelin levels in your blood will result in you wanting to eat more food and, in some cases, particular foods like cake or fries or chocolate.

People who have low ghrelin levels will not eat enough amounts of food and are thus vulnerable to diseases caused by underfeeding. As a corrective measure, such people should receive shots of ghrelin to restore accurate hunger signals in their bodies.

Studies show that obese people suffer from a disconnection between their brains and ghrelin cells, so the blood ghrelin levels go through the roof, which makes these people be in a state of perpetual hunger. So, these obese people respond to their hunger pangs by indulging in their foods of choice, and thus the chronic weight gain becomes hard to manage.

It has been proven that fasting has a positive effect on ghrelin levels. Fasting streamlines the faulty communication between the brain receptors and ghrelin cells. When this is corrected, the brain starts to send out accurate hunger signals, discouraging you from eating more than you should.

- **Increased Lifespan And Slow Aging**

A study by Harvard researchers demonstrated that intermittent fasting led to an increased lifespan and the slowing down of the aging process. These findings were largely hinged on the cell-replenishing effects of fasting and flushing out of toxins.

The average person puts their digestive system under constant load because they're only a short moment away from their next meal. And given the fact that most foods are bacteria-laden, the immune system becomes strained with all the wars that it must be involved in. This makes the body cells prone to accelerated demise. But what happens when you go on a fast?

The energy that would have previously gone into digesting food is used to flush out toxins from the body instead. Also, it has been observed that body cells are strengthened during a fast, which makes physiological functions a bit more robust.

Fasting also enhances the creation of new neural pathways and regeneration of brain cells. This goes towards optimizing the functions of your brain. And, as we know, an energetic brain makes for a "youthful" life.

When you are on a fast, the blood sugar levels are generally down. The skin responds favorably to low blood sugar levels by improving elasticity and keeping wrinkles at bay. A high blood sugar level is notorious for making you ashy and wrinkly.

Fasting may increase your lifespan even from an indirect perspective. For instance, fasting may develop your sense of self-control, improve your discipline, and even increase your creativity. These immaterial resources are very necessary for surviving in the real world.

- **Improved Brain Function**

Fasting triggers the body to destroy its weak cells in a process known as autophagy. One of the main benefits of autophagy is reducing inflammation. Also, autophagy makes way for new and healthy body cells. Autophagy promotes neurogenesis, which is the creation of new brain cells.

Fasting allows the body to deplete the sugars in the blood, and since the body must continue to operate lest it shuts down, the body turns to an alternative energy source: fats. Through the aid of the liver, ketone bodies are produced to supply energy to the brain. Ketone bodies are a much cleaner and reliable source of energy than carbohydrates. Ketone bodies are known to tone down the effects of inflammatory diseases like arthritis.

Fasting promotes high insulin sensitivity. In this way, the body uses less insulin to convert sugars into energy. High insulin sensitivity means that the body will send out accurate signals when it comes to informing the host of either hunger or satiation.

Fasting enhances the production of BDNF (Brain-Derived Neurotrophic Factor), which a plays a critical part in improving neuroplasticity. And thus more resources are committed to the functions of the brain. BDNF is responsible for augmenting areas like memory, learning, and emotions.

Fasting supercharges your mind. It does so through facilitating the creation of new mitochondria. And since mitochondria are the power plants of our bodies, the energy output goes up. This increase in energy and resources causes the brain to function at a much higher level and yields perfect results.

- **Improved Strength And Agility**

When you think of a person that is considered strong and agile, your mind might conceive a well-muscled individual with veins bulging out their neck. Strength and agility come down to practice and more practice. The easiest way to develop agility and strength is obviously through physical training and sticking to a routine until your body adapts.

You must practice every day to be as strong and agile as you'd want to be. Also, you must take particular care over your dietary habits. Professional athletes stick to a diet that has been approved by their doctors for a reason. When it comes to developing strength and agility, nothing matches the combination of exercise and a flawless diet.

But besides fulfilling these two requirements, fasting, too, has its place. Did you know that you can amplify your strength and agility through fasting?

Fasting provokes the body to secrete the Human Growth Hormone. This hormone enhances organ development and even muscle growth. So when you fast, the HGH hormone might be secreted, and it will amplify the effects of your exercise and diet regimen, making you many times stronger and agile.

Fasting will promote the renewal of your body cells and thus lessen the effects of inflammation. When you perform physical exercises, you're basically injuring and damaging your body cells. So, when you fast, you'll allow your body to destroy its weak cells, and make room for new body cells through biogenesis.

Additionally, fasting will go a long way toward improving your motor skills, making you walk with the grace of a cat, with your body parts flexible.

- **Improved Immune System**

The immune system is responsible for defending your body against organisms that are disease vectors. When a foreign organism enters your body, and the body considers it harmful, the immune system immediately comes into action.

Some of the methods suggested for improving the immune system include having a balanced diet, quality sleep, improving your mental health, and taking physical exercises.

Fasting is an understated method of boosting your immune system.

In a research conducted by scientists at the University of Southern California, it emerged that fasting enhanced the rejuvenation of the immune system. Specifically, new white blood cells were formed, strengthening the body's defense system.

The regeneration of the immune system is especially beneficial to people who have a weak body defense mechanism—namely, the elderly, and the sick. This could probably be the reason why an animal in the wild responds to illness by abstaining from food.

In the same study, it was shown that there is a direct correlation between fasting and diminished radical elements in the body. Cell biogenesis was responsible for eradicating inflammation. And moreover, a replenished immune system discouraged the growth of cancer cells.

Depending on how long you observe a fast, the body will, at one point, run out of sugars, and then it will turn to your fat reservoirs to provide energy for its many physiological functions. Fats make for a much cleaner and stable and resourceful energy source than sugars ever will.

So, relying on this fat-energy, the immune system tends to function at a most optimal level.

- **Optimized Physiological Functions**

These are some of the body's physiological functions: sweating, bowel movement, temperature regulation, urinating, and stimuli response.

In a healthy person, all physiological functions should be seamless, but that cannot be said for most of us because our lifestyles get in the way.

So, the next time you rush to the bathroom intending to take a number two only to wind up spending half an hour there, you might want to take a close look at what you are eating.

Fasting is a great method of optimizing your physiological functions. When you observe a normal eating schedule, your body is under constant strain to keep digesting food—a resource-intensive process. But when you go on a fast, the energy that would have been used for digesting food will now be channeled into other critical functions. For instance, the body may now start ridding itself of radicals that promote indigestion, or amp up the blood circulation system, or even devote energy toward enhancing mental clarity, with the result being optimized physiological functions.

With more resources freed up from the strain of digestion, physiological processes will continue seamlessly, and once the glycogen in the blood is over, the body will continue to power physiological functions with energy acquired from fat cells.

The cellular repair benefits attached to fasting enables your body to perform its functions way better. Fasting reduces oxidative stress, which is a key accelerator of aging. In this way, fasting helps restore the youthfulness of your body cells, and the cells are very much optimized for performance.

- **Improved Cardiovascular Health**

When we talk about cardiovascular health, we are essentially talking about the state of the heart, and specifically, its performance in blood circulation.

Factors that improve the condition of your heart include a balanced diet, improved emotional and mental state, quality sleep, and living in a good environment. When cardiovascular health is compromised, it might lead to fatal consequences.

Researchers have long established that fasting improves cardiovascular health.

One of the outcomes of fasting is cholesterol reduction. The lesser cholesterol you have in your blood, the more seamless the movement of blood through your body. Complications are minimal or nonexistent. Thus your heart will be in a great condition.

Fasting also plays a critical role in toning down diabetes. The average diabetic tends to have low insulin sensitivity. For that reason, they need more insulin than is necessary to convert sugars into energy. It puts a strain on body organs and especially the pancreas. This might cause a trickle-down complication that goes back to the heart.

When the body enters fasting mode, it starts using up the stored energy to fulfill other important physiological functions such as blood circulation, in this way boosting the effectiveness of the heart.

Fasting helps you tap into your "higher state." The effects of matured spiritual energy and peaceful inner self cannot be gainsaid. Someone who's at peace with both himself and the universe is bound to develop a very healthy heart, as opposed to one who's constantly bitter, and one who feels as though he's drowning in a bottomless pit.

- **Low Blood Pressure**

People who have a high blood pressure are at risk of damaging not only their heart but their arteries too. When the pressure of the blood flowing in your arteries is high over a long period of time, it is bound to damage the cells of your arteries, and in the worst case scenario, it might trigger a rupture, and cause internal bleeding. High blood pressure puts you at risk of heart failure. Your heart might overwork itself and slowly start wearing out, eventually grinding to a halt.

In people with high blood pressure, a bigger-than-normal left heart is common, and the explanation is that their left heart struggles to maintain the cardiovascular output. So it starts bulking up and eventually creates a disrupting effect on your paired organ. Another risk associated with high blood pressure is coronary disease. This ailment causes your arteries to thin out to the point that it becomes a struggle for blood to flow into your heart. The dangers of coronary disease include arrhythmia, heart failure, and chest pain.

I started by mentioning the risks of high blood pressure because observing a fast normalizes your blood pressure. With a normal blood pressure, you can reverse these risks. Also, normal blood pressure improves the sensitivity of various hormones like ghrelin and leptin, eliminating the communication gap between brain receptors and body cells.

The low blood pressure induced by fasting causes you to have improved motor skills. It is common to hear people admit that fasting makes them feel light and flexible.

- **Decreased Inflammation**

Inflammation is an indication that the body is fighting against an infectious organism. It causes the affected parts to appear red and swollen.

Many diseases that plague us today are rooted in inflammation, and by the look of things, inflammation will be stuck with us for longer than we imagine.

The role of inflammation in mental health cannot be understated. Inflammation is to blame for bad moods, depression, and social anxiety.

The good news though is that fasting can reduce inflammation. Fasting has been shown to be effective in treating mental problems that are rooted in inflammation and as well as safeguarding neural pathways.

Individuals who have incorporated fasting into their lives are much less likely to suffer breakdowns and bad moods than people who don't fast at all.

Asthma, a lung infection, also has an inflammatory background. What's interesting is that fasting alleviates the symptoms of asthma.

The level of hormone sensitivity determines absorption rates of various elements into body cells. For instance, low insulin sensitivity worsens the rate of conversion of sugar into energy. Fasting improves insulin sensitivity, and thus more sugars can be converted into energy.

Fasting enhances the brain to form new pathways when new information is discovered. In this way, your memory power receives a boost, and you are better placed to handle stress and bad thoughts.

Fasting is very efficient in alleviating gut inflammation. Constant fasting promotes healthy gut flora which makes for great bowel movements.

Fasting is a great means of reducing heart inflammation, too. It does so through stabilizing blood pressure and fighting off radical elements.

- **Improved Skin Care**

Most of us are very self-conscious about how we look to the world. Bad skin, acne, and other skin ailments can be a real bother. Fasting has numerous benefits when it comes to improving your skin health, and it is said that fasting bestows a glow on your face. Experts claim that skin ailments develop as a result of terrible stomach environments and that there is a correlation between gut health and skin quality. Fasting promotes the development of gut flora. In this way, your gut health is improved, resulting in improved skin.

When you are on a fast and are taking water, you will eliminate toxins from your body. The condition of your skin improves because the skin cells are free of harmful substances. Many people who previously suffered from a bad skin condition and had tried almost every treatment with no success have admitted that fasting was the only thing that worked.

Another benefit of fasting is that it slows down the aging process. The water consumed during the fast goes to flush out toxins, consequently reducing the effects of old age on your skin. Fasting also promotes low blood sugar. Low blood sugar promotes optimized physiological processes and, as a result, toning down the effects of aging.

When you go on a fast, the body allocates energy to areas that might have previously been overlooked. So, your bad skin condition may be treated with the stored up energy, and considering that the energy produced from fat is more stable and resourceful; your skin health will improve.

- **Autophagy**

This is the process whereby the body rids itself of weakened and damaged cells. Autophagy is triggered by dry fasting. The body simply "eats" the weakened cells to provide water to the healthy cells. Eliminated cells are usually weak and damaged. And their absence creates room for new cells that are obviously going to be powerful.

Autophagy has been shown to have many benefits, and they include:

- **Slowing down aging effects**

The formation of wrinkles and body deterioration are some of the effects of aging. However, thanks to autophagy, these effects can be reversed, since the body will destroy its old and weakened cells and replace them with new cells.

- **Reducing inflammation**

Inflammation is responsible for many diseases affecting us today, but thanks to autophagy, the cells that have been affected by inflammation are consumed, giving room for new cells.

- **Conserving energy**

Autophagy elevates the body into a state of energy conservation. In this way, your body can utilize resources in a most careful manner.

- **Fighting infections**

The destruction of old and weak body cells creates room for fresh and powerful body cells. In that vein, old and weakened white blood cells are destroyed, and then new powerful white blood cells are formed. These new white new blood cells fortify the immune system.

- **Improving motor skills**

Autophagy plays a critical role in improving the motor skills of an individual. This goes toward boosting the strength and agility of a person. Energy drawn from the weak and damaged cells is way more resourceful than the energy drawn from sugars.

Summary

There are numerous benefits attached to fasting. One of them is increased insulin sensitivity. When the insulin sensitivity goes up, insulin resistance drops, and the body is now able to use less insulin to convert sugars into energy. Another benefit of fasting is improved leptin sensitivity. The leptin hormone is known as the satiation hormone, and it is responsible for alerting you when you are full. An improved ghrelin level is another benefit of fasting. The ghrelin hormone is known as the hunger hormone. It induces hunger pangs so that you may feed. Fasting lengthens your existence. This is largely because of neuroregeneration of cells and flushing out toxins. Fasting improves brain function, strengthens your body and boosts agility, strengthens your immune system, optimizes your physiological functions, improves cardiovascular health, lowers blood pressure, reduces inflammation, improves your skin, and promotes autophagy. As researchers carry out new experiments, more benefits of fasting are being uncovered.

Chapter 4: Myths and Dangers of Fasting

Long-Held Myths and Misconceptions about Fasting

Fasting has gained widespread acceptance across the world. More people who are seeking to improve their health through alternative means are turning to fasting. As you might expect, the field has been marred with conspiracies, lies, half-truths, and outright ignorance. Some of the long-held myths and misconceptions about fasting include:

Fasting makes you overeat. This myth hinges on the idea that after observing a fast, an individual is bound to be so hungry that they will consume more food to compensate for the period they'd abstained from food.

The brain requires a steady supply of sugars. Some people say that the brain cannot operate normally in the absence of sugars. These people believe that the brain uses sugars alone to power its activities and any other source of energy would not be compatible. So when you fast, you'd be risking shutting down your brain functions.

Skipping breakfast will make you fat. Some people seem to treat breakfast as though it were an unexplained mystery of the Earth. They say breakfast is special. Anyone who misses breakfast cannot possibly have a healthy life. They say that if you skip breakfast, you will be under a heavy spell of cravings, and finally give in to unhealthy foods.

Fasting promotes eating disorders. Some people seem to think that fasting is the stepping stone for disorders like bulimia and anorexia. They complain that once you see the effects of fasting, you might want to "amplify" the effects which might make you susceptible to an eating disorder like anorexia.

Busting Myths Associated with Fasting

Fasting will make you overeat. This is partly true. However, it is important to note that most people fall into the temptation of overeating because of their lack of discipline and not necessarily because of unrealistic demands of fasting. If you're fasting the proper way, no temptation is big enough to lead you astray, and after all, the temptation exists to test whether you're really disciplined.

The brain requires a steady supply of sugars. This myth perpetuates the notion that we should consume carbohydrates every now and again to keep the brain in working condition. Also, this myth suggests that the brain can only use energy derived from sugars and not energy derived from fats. When you go on a fast, and your body uses up all the glycogen, your liver produces ketone bodies that are passed on to your brain to act as an energy source.

Skipping breakfast will make you fat. There is nothing special about breakfast. You can decide to skip breakfast and adhere to your schedule and be able to get desired results. It's true that skipping breakfast will cause you to be tempted by cravings, but you're not supposed to give in, and in that case, you become the problem. Skipping breakfast will not make you fat. What will make you fat is you pouring more calories into your body than you will spend.

Fasting promotes eating disorders. If you have a goal in mind, you are supposed to stay focused on that goal. The idea that an individual would plunge into the world of eating disorders simply because they want to amplify the results of fasting sounds like weakness on the part of the individual and not a fault of the practice itself.

Dangers of Fasting

Just as with most things in life, there's both a positive and negative side to fasting. Most of these problems are amplified in people who either fast in the wrong way or people who clearly shouldn't be fasting.

So let's explore some of the risks that are attached to fasting.

- **Dehydration**

Chances are, you will suffer dehydration while observing a fast, and drinking regular cups of water won't make the situation any better. Well, this is because most of your water intake comes from the foods that you consume daily. When dehydration kicks in, you are bound to experience nausea, headaches, constipation, and dizziness.

- **Orthostatic Hypotension**

This is common in people who drink water during their fasts. Orthostatic Hypotension causes your body to react unfavorably when you move around. For instance, when you stand on your feet and walk around, you might experience dizziness and feel as though you're at the verge of blowing up into smithereens. Other symptoms include temporary mental blindness, lightheadedness, and vision problems. These symptoms make it hard for you to function in activities that demand precision and focus, e.g., driving.

- **Worsened medical conditions**

People who fast while they are sick put themselves at risk of worsening their condition. The fast may amplify the symptoms of their diseases. People with the following ailments should first seek doctor's approval before getting into fasting: gout, type 2 diabetes, chronic kidney disease, eating disorders, and heartburn.

- **Increased stress**

The habit of skipping meals might lead to increased stress. The body might respond to hunger by increasing the hormone cortisol which is responsible for high-stress levels. And when you are in a stressed mental state, it becomes difficult to function in your day to day life.

Summary
Although fasting has a lot of benefits, there is a dark side to it too, but the negative effects can be minimized or eliminated altogether when a

professional is involved. Dehydration is one of the negative effects. Besides providing nutrients to the body, food is also an important source of water. So when you fail to correct this gap by drinking a lot more water, your body will fall into a state of dehydration. Orthostatic hypotension is another danger. This illness makes you feel dizzy and lightheaded, and so it makes it difficult for you to function in an activity that demands your focus and stamina. Fasting may amplify the symptoms of your disease depending on your age and the stage of your disease. For instance, people who suffer from illnesses like gout, diabetes, eating disorders, and heartburn should first seek the doctor's approval before going on a fast. Moreover, fasting may lead to an increase in stress levels.

Chapter 5: Safety, Side Effects, and Warning

As the subject of fasting becomes popular, more people are stating their opinions on it, and as you might expect, some people are for it, and others are against it.

The best approach toward fasting is not set in stone, but it is rather determined by factors such as your age and health status.

Before you get into fasting, there are some critical balances you need to consider first. One of them is your experience. If you have never attempted a fast before, then it is a bad idea to go straight into a 48-hour fast, because you are likely to water down the effects. As a beginner, you must always start with lighter fasts and build your way up into extended fasts. You could begin by skipping one meal, then two meals, and finally the whole day.

Another important metric when it comes to determining the appropriate space between your eating windows is your health status. For instance, you cannot be a sufferer of late-stage malaria and yet go on a fast, because it might create a multiplying effect on your symptoms. People who are malnourished or have eating disorders might want to find other ways of improving their health apart from fasting.

An essential thing to note is that we are not all alike. My body's response to a fast is not going to be the exact response of yours. Knowing this, always listen to your body. Sometimes, a water-fast might trigger a throat infection and make your throat swollen. In such a situation, it would be prudent to suspend the fast and take care of your throat, as opposed to sticking to your guns.

Side Effects of Fasting

Fasting might upset the physiological functions of a body. This explains the side effects that crop up when you go on a fast. It is also important to note that most of these side effects subside as your body grows accustomed to the fast.

- **Cravings**

Top on the list is cravings. When you go on a fast, the immediate response by the body is to elevate the "hunger hormone" and so, you will start craving for sweet unhealthy foods. If you are not the disciplined type, this is a huge pitfall that could negate the effects of your fast.

- **Headaches**

Headaches, too, are a side effect of fasting. Most people who are new to fasting are bound to experience a headache. One of the explanations for headaches is that it is the brain's response to a shift from relying on carbohydrates to ketone bodies as the alternative energy source. Regular consumption of water might mitigate the headache or eliminate it altogether.

- **Low energy**

Another side effect is low energy. When you fast, the body might interpret it as starving, and its first response will be conserving energy. So, there will be less energy for physiological functions. In this way, you will start feeling less energetic than before.

- **Irritability**

Irritability is also a side effect. Studies show that people who are new to fasting are bound to have foul moods as their body increases stress hormones and hunger hormones. However, if they can persist, the irritability will eventually go away, and make room for a happy mood as the body switches to its fat stores for energy.

Types of People That Should Not Fast

The ideal person to go on a fast is a healthy person. People with certain medical conditions may still go on a fast, but it is always prudent to seek the guidance of a medical professional. We have previously stated that fasting strengthens the immune system. So is it contradicting to discourage fasting when one is sick? No! You may fast but preferably under the instruction and supervision of a medical professional. However, there are cases when it is inappropriate to fast.

Infants and children. Putting kids on a fast is just wrong. Their bodies are not fully developed yet to withstand periods of hunger. Fasting would do them more damage than good. For instance, it might mess with their metabolism and have a negative impact on their growth curve.

Hypoglycemics. People with hypoglycemia have extremely low levels of blood sugar. Their bodies need a constant stream of sugars to sustain normal functions lest severe illnesses take reign. For that reason, hypoglycemics should not fast.

Pregnant and nursing women. These women need a lot of energy because their young ones are dependent on them. So, pregnant women and nursing women are encouraged to keep their blood sugar steady.

The malnourished. People who are underweight and malnourished should stay away from fasting. To start with, their bodies don't have sufficient fat. So, when they go on a fast, their body will destroy its cells in search of nutrients. Over time, the results could be fatal.

People with heartburn. People who experience severe heartburn should not fast. This is because heartburn is a very distressing thing and there is no guarantee it will subside even when your body adapts to fasting. So, it is better to stay clear.

Impaired immune system. Fasting may have the ability to renew the strength and utility of your immune system. But when we are talking about an impaired immune system where most of the white blood cells are hanging on a thin blade, then fasting cannot be of help. Such a person would be better off sticking to a healthy diet.

Other classes of people that shouldn't fast include those recovering from surgeries, people with eating disorders, depressed souls, and people with extreme heart disease.

Summary

For purposes of safety, always ensure that your body is prepared to withstand the effects of fasting. You may prepare by evaluating your health status, experience, and developing a great sense of self-awareness. Fasting may have its numerous benefits, but there is also a negative side to it because fasting comes with unpleasant side effects. The good thing though is that most of these side effects tend to subside once the body grows accustomed to your fasting routine. One of the side effects of fasting is getting a headache. A headache is triggered by the brain's adjustment from relying on carbohydrates as an energy source and switching to ketone bodies. It may be mitigated through constant consumption of water. Another side effect is cravings. Your body makes you want to eat fast foods very badly. Fasting may also make you irritable, but it is for only a short time and then a happy mood sets in. Fasting also makes you feel less energetic, which can be uninspiring. These are some of the people that shouldn't fast: hypoglycemics, infants, children, pregnant women, nursing women, the malnourished, people with extreme ailments, and those recovering from surgeries.

Chapter 6: Intermittent Fasting

What Is Intermittent Fasting?

Nowadays, intermittent fasting is one of the most talked about practices in health improvement domains. Basically, intermittent fasting is about creating a routine where you eat only after a set period of time. Intermittent fasting has been shown to have numerous benefits such as improving motor skills, developing willpower, and brain functions. Most people are turning to the practice to achieve their health goals—specifically, weight loss.

The most common way of performing an intermittent fast is by skipping meals. In the beginning, you may decide to skip one of the main meals, and when your body adapts to two meals a day, you may then elevate to just one meal per day. During the fast, you are not supposed to partake of any food, but it is okay to drink water and other low-calorie drinks like black coffee or black tea.

Intermittent fasting allows you to indulge in the foods of your choice, but there's emphasis on avoiding foods that are traditionally bad for your health. The main thing is to give your body time to process food between your eating windows.

Polls answered by people who have adopted this lifestyle indicate that most of them are happy with the results. Intermittent fasting is a very effective means of weight loss as it improves the metabolic rate of the body, as well as triggers cell autophagy. The good thing about intermittent fasting is that it allows you to partake of your favorite foods without making you feel guilty, which is a contrast to fad diets that insist on eating things like raw food and plant-based foods.

How to Practice Intermittent Fasting

There are a couple of ways to practice intermittent fasting. These are the three most popular ways:

That's counterproductive. Make sure you have some experience before you fast for an extended period of time.

You'll find that what works for someone won't necessarily work for everybody else. So what's one supposed to do? Test, test, test. At one point you will find a variation of the intermittent fast that will fit perfectly into your life. It's all about finding what really works for you and then committing to the routine.

In my experience, I have found the 16:8 to be the best. This type of intermittent fast requires that you abstain from food for 16 hours and then indulge for 8 hours. For most followers of this routine, they like to have their eating window between 12:00 PM and 20:00 PM. The 16-hour fast will be inclusive of sleep, which makes it less severe.

This method is extremely efficient in weight loss, and most people have reported success. However, you must stick to the routine for a while before you can see any results. Don't do it for just one day and climb on the weighing machine only to find that there are no changes and then give up.

To improve the success of fasting intermittently, stick to a balanced diet during your eating windows, and don't take the fast as an excuse for indulging in unhealthy foods.

Step-By-Step Process of Fasting For a Week

The first step is to certify that you are in perfect condition. Get an appointment with your doctor and perform a whole health analysis to get a clean bill of health. Remember to always start with a small fast and gradually build up.

- **Day one**

When you wake up, forgo breakfast and opt for a glass of water or black coffee. Then go on about your work as you normally do. Around noon, your eating window opens. Now you are free to indulge in the food of your choice, but make sure that they are nutritious foods because unhealthy foods will water down your efforts. Your eating window should close at 20:00 PM, and from 20:01 pm to 12:00 pm the next day, don't consume anything else besides water.

- **Day two**

On day two, your body should have started to protest over the sudden calorie reduction, and so you'll be likely experiencing an irritable mood, lightheadedness, and a small headache. When you wake up, no matter how strong the urge to eat might be, just push it back, and the only thing you should consume is water or black coffee. At noon, your eating window opens, and you're free to eat until 8 pm.

- **Day three**

When you wake up, take a glass of water or black coffee. Chances are that your body has started to adjust to the reduced daily caloric intake. It has switched to burning fats. At twelve noon, when your eating window opens, consume less food than you did yesterday and the day before, so that the body has even lesser calories to work with. The body should adapt to this pretty swiftly.

- **Day four**

In the morning, take a glass of water or black coffee and go about your business. When your eating window opens, eat as much food as you ate yesterday, but in the evening, resist the urge to drink anything.

- **Day five**

When you wake up, take a glass of water or black coffee. During your eating window, eat less food than you did previously. At night, resist the urge to drink water.

- **Day six**

When you wake up, resist the urge to drink water or even coffee. In your eating window, choose not to eat at all, and at night give in to the temptation and drink water or black coffee.

- **Day seven**

When you wake up, take a glass of water or black coffee. In your eating window, resume eating, but only take a small portion, and just before you close the eating window, eat again, except it should be a slightly larger meal than previously. Before you sleep, take another glass of water or black coffee. Fast till your next eating window, and then you may resume your normal eating habits. At this point, you will have lost weight and experienced a host of other benefits attached to intermittent fasting.

Summary

Intermittent fasting features a cycle of fasting interrupted by an eating window. Some of the methods of intermittent fasting include the 16:8, eat-stop-eat, 5:2, and alternate-day fasting. The best approach to intermittent fasting is context-based in the sense that only you can know what works for you. The most popular form of intermittent fasting is the 16:8. In this method, you fast for 16 hours and then an eating window of 8 hours. The biggest advantage of intermittent fasting is that it announces relief to your pocket. The "food budget" goes into other uses. The amount of time that it takes to prepare meals is a real hassle, but intermittent fasting frees up your time so you can be more productive. The entry barrier is nonexistent too. This means anyone can practice intermittent fasting because there are no barriers or things to buy—a stark contrast to other weight loss methods like fad diets that may be both inconveniencing and expensive.

Chapter 7: Longer Periods of Fasting

Fasting for longer periods is reserved for people who have a bit of experience with fasting. A newbie shouldn't get into it.

It is basically desisting from food for not less than 24 hours, but not more than, say, 48 hours. You may increase the success of the fast by making it a dry fast. In a dry fast, you won't have the luxury of drinking water or any other low-calorie drink like black coffee.

Fasting for longer periods requires that you prepare emotionally, mentally, and physically. The buildup to your fast is an especially important part. Your food consumption should be minimal.

Fasting for a longer period helps you achieve much more results because the body will be subjected to an increased level of strain.

However, you must take care to know when to stop. In some instances, the body might rebel by either catching an infection or shutting down critical functions, and in such times it is prudent to call off the fast.

During longer fasts, you should abstain from strenuous exercises, because the body will be in a state of energy conservation, and the available energy is purposed for physiological functions.

With the wrong approach, long fasts might become disastrous. That's why it is always important to seek clearance from your doctor first before you go into the fast. And to flush out toxins, ensure you have a steady intake of water.

It is estimated that weight loss in longer fasts averages around one to two pounds every day.

How to Fast for Longer Periods
The main reason that people go into longer fasts is to obviously lose

weight. But you might want to fast to reach other purposes such as flushing toxins from your body or heightening your mental capabilities. Also, a longer fast is recommended if you are going into a surgery.

The response to a fast is different for everyone. If it is your first time, please take great care by getting medical clearance.

As your fast approaches, you might want to minimize your food consumption to get used to managing hunger.

Next, you should clear away items that might ruin your focus or tempt you to backslide. You might want to give your kitchen a total makeover by, for instance, clearing away the bad food. It is much easier to manage cravings when they are out of sight than when they are within easy reach.

Always start small. Before you deprive yourself food for over 24 hours, you should first get a taste of what food deprivation for 8 hours feels like, and if you can handle that, then you're ready to step up your game. While you fast, you should be very aware of the ranges of effects that your body experiences. You might feel dizzy, lightheaded, sleepy, or distressed, and these are okay reactions. Things that are not okay are infections and prolonged aches of body parts. If your body responds to fasting unfavorably, you should stop the fast.

Pros and Cons of Fasting for Longer Periods

If you have always been motivated to clear away the stubborn fat in your body, but have never found an efficient method, then the answer is to fast for a longer period.

When you go on a longer fast, the body uses up all glycogen in the first 24 hours, and then it switches to burning fats. A longer fast guarantees quick weight loss.

A longer fast saves you money. Food is an expensive affair, especially if you eat out. With a longer fast, it means you are staying away from food, and are thus saving on food costs.

Besides the benefit of optimizing your health, a longer fast will strengthen both your willpower and mental sharpness, which are two necessary factors in attaining success.

Fasting for a longer period helps you appreciate the taste of food. By the time you're done fasting, you'll want to indulge your appetite, and food will suddenly taste so sweet. The scarcity factor elevates the value of food.

A longer fast has cons, too. One of the biggest cons is the strain that it puts on your body. When your body goes from relying on glycogen into fats as a source of energy, nasty side effects are bound to come up—for instance, headaches, nausea, and lightheadedness.

Another con is that fasting for a longer period might open you up to disease. As much as fasting renews your immune system, your body still needs robust energy to function optimally. Fasting puts your body into a state of conserving energy which makes it easy for disease to attack.

Step-By-Step Process of Fasting for Longer Periods
When you decide to go on a fast for a longer period, you must realize that you are signing up for a real challenge. The body's immediate response to a fast is raising the hunger hormone to alert you to look for food. Now, fighting off that urge takes a lot of willpower. In some regard, it's why fasting might be considered a test of discipline because not so many people can withstand it.

So here's the step-by-step process of going on a fast for longer periods:

Preparation
The first major thing is to ensure that your body is in a condition that will allow you to fast, without any complications. In other words, consult your

doctor for a checkup.

Reduce your food intake in the days leading up to your fast so that your body can get accustomed to staying without food. Once your body is familiar with the feeling of food deprivation, you are ready to move forward.

In the morning of your fast, drink lots of water. It is critical for flushing out toxins and reducing stomach acidity when your stomach secretes acids in anticipation of food. Your water intake should be regular and spread out through the day.

Rather than lying down and wearing a look of self-pity, just go on about your work as you normally would, provided it is not a very focus-oriented job like performing surgeries.

You should stay the whole day without food and then go to bed. On the following morning, your hunger pangs will be even more amplified, at which point you are to mitigate the hunger with a drink of water and then maintain the fast for another 24 hours. 48 hours are enough for a longer fast, and the weight loss should be dramatic. After the fast, don't immediately go back to eating heavy amounts of food, but rather ease your way into a lighter diet.

Chapter 8: Extended Fasting

Fasting for an extended period is an extreme form of fasting that demands you abstain from food from anywhere between three days to seven days. If you can deny yourself food for more than three days, you should be proud of yourself, because not so many people have that kind of determination.

Fasting for an extended period of time amplifies the results of a longer fast. When you go for an extended period of time without food, you will allow yourself to experience a range of different feelings. At the initial stage there is distress, and towards the end your feelings become tranquil.

Considering that this is an especially long fast, you are supposed to take a very keen listen to the response by your body. If your body sends out the message that it is under massive strain, now it's time to stop the fast. Cases where it's appropriate to stop include developing stomach ulcers, throat infection, and loss of consciousness.

You should eat lighter meals as you approach the start of your fast. During the fast, your water intake should be regular. When you complete the fast, the transition to your normal eating life should be slow and gradual, starting with lighter meals.

Fasting for an extended period has the biggest potential of going wrong. The prolonged food deprivation in itself may do more good than harm. There is also the possibility of slightly altering your body's physiological functions. Still, the benefits of an extended fast outweigh the negatives.

Pros and Cons of Fasting for Extended Periods
The biggest advantage of fasting for an extended period of time is the discipline it instills in you. When you go for a prolonged period without

eating food, your body will respond by increasing hunger pangs. It takes extreme willpower to keep going. This experience can help you build your self-control and discipline in real life.

An extended fast is very effective in banishing stubborn fat. Most people who are obese will tell you that they are trying to lose weight, but the fat is stubborn. Guess what, their methods are ineffective. However, if they had the will and courage to go on an extended fast, then they'd experience a rapid weight loss and reach their desired weight.

Extended fasting promotes a high rate of cell replenishing. When the body goes for days without food, it turns in on itself and begins to digest its cells—the weak and damaged cells—to provide nutrition for the healthy cells. The elimination of weak and damaged cells creates room for new and healthy ones.

The biggest disadvantage for an extended period of fasting is the risk of complications that you put your body into. Some complications might be instant whereas others may develop long after the fast. The biggest risk is catching an infection. If you're unlucky enough that you catch some disease in your fast, your immune system will be overwhelmed.

Another huge miss about extended fasting is the disconnect it encourages in your normal life. When you are fasting, you won't be able to share a meal with your friends or family, and that can be a big inconvenience. It can make people "talk."

Step-By-Step Process of Fasting for Extended Periods

When you get clearance from a medical professional, you should start by preparing for the extended fast. Ideally, if you are getting into an extended fast, you should have experience with either intermittent fasting, longer fasting or both. The more your body is familiar with food deprivation, the better the outcome.

On the start of your extended fast, you should consume only water or black coffee, and throughout the rest of the day, observe regular water consumption. It will aid in flushing out toxins and other harmful elements from your body.

During the fast, you should keep your normal work schedule, as opposed to being inactive, because inactivity will worsen your hunger pangs. The standard response to hunger pangs should be water consumption.

On the second day, first thing in the morning is to consume more water. This water is very critical in flushing out toxins and keeping your body cells hydrated as well as regulating autophagy. However, if you want to increase the success rate of the fast, you might consider eliminating water. One of the side effects of this type of fast is a dry mouth. A dry mouth has the potential of being very distressing. For purposes of safety, always hydrate yourself.

On the third day, wake up and consume water or black coffee. At this point, your body is subsisting on its fat reserves, and the weight loss is evident. Your body has potentially minimized hunger pangs to manageable levels. Keep yourself busy. Otherwise, inactivity will provoke hunger.

From the fourth day up until the seventh, keep the same routine. When you come to the end of your fast, realize that your body will be in starvation mode, so don't immediately consume large amounts of food. Instead, ease your way back into a normal eating schedule.

Chapter 9: The Eating Window

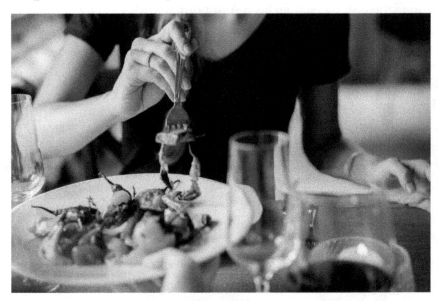

What is the Eating Window?

The eating window is the period of time that you are allowed to indulge in foods and one that precedes a period of fasting. The eating window comes around on a cycle, and you should adhere to it by only eating when the window opens and abstaining from food the rest of the time.

The hours are not set in stone. You are free to choose your eating window in a way that works for you. Most people who practice intermittent fasting seem to adhere to an eight-hour eating window followed by a sixteen-hour fast. Commonly, the eight-hour window opens at around 12:00 PM and goes all the way to 20:00 PM. During this time, you may indulge in your favorite foods. However, past 20:00 PM, you are supposed to observe the fast.

The 16:8 method of intermittent fasting appeals to many people because the 16 hours of fasting are inclusive of the bed-time. If you are not into waiting for sixteen hours before you partake of food, you may lessen the hours, so that you will have frequent eating windows between your fasts.

It is generally more fruitful to have a small eating window followed by a long period of fast.

It's also important to choose an eating window that optimizes your health. For instance, eating during the day is of much benefit than eating at night. This is because the body puts more calories to use during the day as opposed to while you are asleep. Also, adhere to a good diet, or else your gains will be neutralized by a bad diet.

What to Eat

The reason why intermittent fasting appeals to so many people is the nonexistent dietary rules common in alternative weight loss methods like fad diets. In intermittent fasting, you are free to eat the foods of your choice, and the main thing is to restrict your caloric intake.

You are free to consume the foods that delight you, but be careful not to fall in the pit of overcompensation. You are at risk of misleading yourself into consuming unhealthy foods during your eating window under the delusion that fasting will take care of it. Truth is, some of the fast foods we indulge are so calorie-laden that it would take a prolonged fast (not intermittent) to eliminate their fat from our bodies.

Limit your intake of red meat. As much as intermittent fasting is lenient when it comes to diet, it is widely known that red meat causes more harm than good. So, you might want to limit its intake or eliminate it altogether.

Fruits are a source of essential nutrients for the body. Always make sure to include fruits like bananas, avocados, and apples into your meals. Fruits help reduce inflammation and are critical in optimizing the physiological functions of the body.

Vegetables should be in your meals. People who claim that vegetables taste bad are just unimaginative cooks. Vegetables do taste good. And some of the health benefits of vegetable include strengthening your bones, stabilizing your blood sugar, boosting your brain health, and improving your digestive system.

Developing Discipline

It takes a lot of discipline to persevere through a fast. Think about it. The average person is accustomed to eating something every now and then. They cannot afford to hold back for even a couple more hours when lunch is due. The eating cycle never ends. And so a person who can decide to abstain from food and stick to their decision is a special kind of person—he/she is disciplined.

The biggest challenge when it comes to fasting for an extended period is to overcome the hunger pangs over the first few days. Your body floods you with the hunger hormone, pushing you to look for food. However, if you persevere through the first few days, your body will adjust to the food deprivation and switch to your stored fats as the alternative source of energy.

One of the things you must do to boost your self-control is to prepare your mind. When you have an idea of what to expect, the hunger will be more tolerable as opposed to if you're ignorant. Another thing to take into consideration is the weather. You don't want to fast during a cold season because fasting lowers your body temperature, and so you'll be hard-hit.

Another way of boosting your discipline is joining hands with people of the same goal. In this way, you can keep each other in check. When you are on a team or have a friend who practices fasting too, it will be easy to stick to your plan, as everybody will offer psycho-social support to everybody else. Sometimes, the difference between throwing in the towel and sticking to your guns is a kind word of encouragement.

Summary

The eating window is the period of time that you are allowed to indulge in foods and one that precedes a period of fasting. The eating window comes around on a cycle, and you should adhere to it by only eating when the window opens and abstaining from food the rest of the time. Intermittent fasting doesn't restrict the consumption of certain foods as is common for other weight loss methods such as fad diets. To boost the effectiveness of your fast, your diet should be balanced, which means it should include foods rich in minerals and vitamins. There also should be fruits and vegetables. Discipline is very important when it comes to fasting. It's what keeps you going when your body protests hunger. The most important step toward developing discipline is to first prepare mentally for the fast. Another way of developing discipline is by having a strong support system

Chapter 10: Fasting For Weight Loss

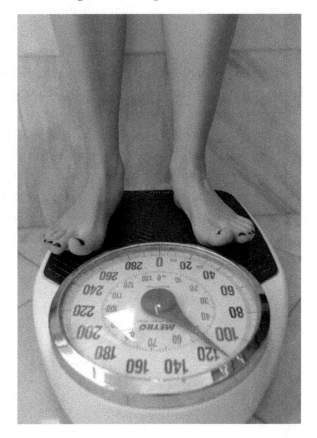

Why You'll Lose Weight through Fasting

Some of the methods of losing weight include fad diets, exercising, and supplements. However, these methods are not very effective, and in most cases, they cannot solve obesity on their own.

Fasting is easily the best method of not only reducing weight but also eliminating the stubborn lower-stomach fat. But why is it so?

First off, fasting optimizes the biological functions of your body. Fasting allows you to ease the load on your digestive system. The spare energy goes toward optimizing your physiological functions. For instance, improved digestion streamlines your bowel movement too. This efficacy in the physiological functions creates a compounding effect that leads to the shedding of dead weight, thus reducing an individual's weight and actually stabilizing it.

Another way in which fasting promotes weight loss is through cell autophagy. A dry fast is particularly what triggers cell autophagy. When the body uses up all its water, it now starts digesting the weak and damaged cells to provide water for the body cells that are in a much better state. Autophagy helps in eliminating dead and weak cells thereby making a person lighter.

Fasting plays a critical role in improving the metabolic health of an individual. With improved metabolism, the body can crunch more calories, and thus the individual's weight goes down.

Fasting improves insulin sensitivity. This helps the body to convert more sugars into energy. The body uses more calories, and as a result, there's a loss of weight.

In most obese people, the communication between their brain and ghrelin cells is warped, which makes them experience hunger all the time, even when they are full. Fasting helps remedy this problem, and obese people start receiving accurate signals when they are hungry.

Step-By-Step Process of Losing Weight through Fasting

- **Checkup**

First off, make sure that your body is in a condition that allows you to fast. Some of the people who are discouraged from the practice include pregnant women, nursing women, infants, sufferers of late-stage terminal illnesses, and those who are recovering from surgery.

- **Water**

Your body will respond to food deprivation by secreting acids and enzymes, and for that reason, always start your fast with consuming water. Regular water consumption will flush out the toxins and will also ease you from stomach pain.

- **Eating window**

Desist from food for at least 16 hours and then take a meal of your choice. The ideal eating window should be around eight hours. During this eight hour break, you are free to indulge. However, you must take care not to consume unhealthy foods. They will just neutralize your fasting efforts. Also, mind the portions. Simply because you have eight hours to feed doesn't mean you should fill up that period with food only.

- **Exercise**

Taking aerobic exercises, in particular, will have a dramatic effect on your weight loss. Aerobic exercises act like a calorie furnace. Also, exercises will increase the toxins in your body, and for that reason, keep yourself hydrated.

- **Breaking the fast**

At the end of your fast, never go right back into "heavy eating," but rather ease your way back by first consuming lighter foods. It'd be prudent of you to make fasting a part of your lifestyle. The key thing is to go with works for you. Most people seem to prefer intermittent fasting because it can fit in most people's lives. Prolonged fasting should be done sparingly as it carries the risk of developing complications.

Summary

Fasting has a positive impact on the rate of metabolism. When the metabolism rate is high, the energy output of the body goes up, and thus more calories are used up. This creates a caloric deficit and subsequent weight loss. Fasting promotes cell autophagy. Autophagy is the process where weak and damaged body cells are digested by the body. The elimination of weak body cells helps in weight reduction. High insulin resistance makes it hard for the body cells to absorb the sugars in the blood. But fasting reduces insulin resistance so that the body will use less insulin to convert sugars into energy. Before you go on a fast, you should get medical clearance. Some of the people who shouldn't get into a fast include the terminally ill, pregnant women, nursing women, and people who are recovering from surgery. It is important to take water throughout the fast to flush out toxins and mitigate the effect of stomach acids.

Chapter 11: Fasting for Type 2 Diabetes

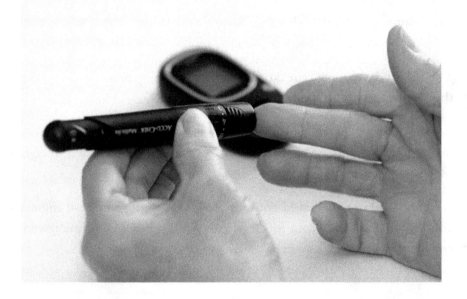

What is Type 2 Diabetes?

Type 2 diabetes is a disease that damages the ability of the pancreas to produce sufficient insulin. Insulin is the hormone produced by the pancreas, and its main function is to regulate the conversion of glucose into energy. The body cells of people who have type 2 diabetes are insensitive to insulin, and as such, they experience difficulty in converting sugars into energy. This condition is known as insulin resistance. It is characterized by the production of higher amounts of insulin, but the body cannot absorb it.

As to the origin of type 2 diabetes, scientists have established that it is genetic. The disease is handed down to progeny. Another leading cause of type 2 diabetes is obesity. Overweight people are much more likely to develop insulin resistance. There's a link between childhood obesity and development of type 2 diabetes in adulthood.

Another contributing factor is a metabolic syndrome. High insulin resistance is a result of increased blood pressure and cholesterol. Excessive sugars produced by the liver may also be a trigger.

The symptoms of type 2 diabetes cover a wide range. They include thirst, frequent peeing, hazy vision, irritability, tiredness, and yeast infections.

The risk of developing type 2 diabetes can be greatly minimized by taking the following actions:

Losing weight. Weight loss improves insulin sensitivity, and thus the buildup of insulin in the blood is eliminated. Also, there's more conversion of sugars into energy.

Balanced diet. You should consume foods that are sources of minerals and vitamins. Increase your intake of fruits and vegetables. Minimize your consumption of sugars and red meat.

The Role of Insulin in the Body

The insulin hormone is produced by the pancreas. Its key role is to regulate blood sugar. Increased insulin resistance might lead to type 2 diabetes. Insulin plays the critical role of facilitating absorption of sugars into body cells. In this way, insulin helps to reduce the blood sugar level. Another important role of insulin is to modify the activity of enzymes. The enzymes are secreted by the body when there's food in the stomach. Insulin regulates the activity of enzymes.

Insulin helps the body recover quickly. When your body is recovering from an injury or illness, insulin plays a critical role in speeding up the healing process by transporting amino acids to cells.

Insulin promotes gut flora and thus improves gut health. This improves bowel movement. Insulin also improves the excretion of harmful substances like sodium.

Insulin promotes brain health. It improves brain clarity by providing the essential nutrients to the brain.

Insulin plays a key role in determining the metabolism rate of the body. In instances of high insulin sensitivity, the blood glucose is easily absorbed into the cells, making for a high metabolic rate. But in instances of low insulin sensitivity, the process of converting sugars into energy becomes hard, and, consequently, there is a low metabolic rate.

Insulin is very important in the optimal functioning of your body. Some of the factors that improve the production of the insulin hormone are having a balanced diet, improving your brain health, having quality sleep, exercising, and staying in a pollution-free environment.

How Diabetes Affects both Production and Usage of Insulin

Diabetes is a major lifestyle disease all over the world. A person who has diabetes either cannot produce sufficient insulin, or their body cells are insensitive to insulin. Diabetes is broadly classified into two types: type 1 and type 2.

People who suffer from type 1 diabetes produce little to no insulin. This slows down the rate of conversion of sugars into energy. A low level of insulin is mainly a result of the immune system attacking the pancreas and curtailing its ability to produce sufficient insulin. Also, low insulin levels might be a result of weakened and damaged body cells. Type 1 diabetes commonly affects young people. One of the corrective measures is to administer insulin through injections.

Symptoms of type 1 diabetes include dehydration, constant urge to urinate, hunger (even after eating), unexplained weight loss, blurry vision, exhaustion, and bad moods.

Type 2 diabetes is the most common form of diabetes. People who suffer from type 2 diabetes have a high insulin resistance. Their body cells are averse to insulin. Types 2 diabetes is treated by increasing insulin sensitivity.

Symptoms of type 2 diabetes include tiredness, never-ending thirst, constant urge to pee, irritability, weak immune, and shivering.

The pancreas is the organ that produces insulin. When we consume food, blood sugar rises. The pancreas releases insulin to facilitate the conversion of sugars into energy. But someone who suffers from diabetes either lacks sufficient insulin or their body cannot use the released insulin. This results in increased blood sugar levels. This scenario presents risks such as the development of heart disease and stroke.

How Blood Sugar Responds To Fasting
A carbohydrate metabolism test is crucial in determining how blood sugar responds to fasting. The test is conducted on diabetics. During a fast, the levels of plasma glucose go up. People with diabetes either cannot produce sufficient insulin, or their bodies are resistant to insulin. Non-diabetics, though, produce insulin that brings down the levels of glucose through absorption.

Diet greatly affects the blood sugar rate-of-increase. For instance, a big serving of food will trigger a high level of blood sugar, and sugar-laden foods like cake, bread, and fries will also increase the blood sugar level.

People with type 1 diabetes lack sufficient insulin because their immune system attacks the pancreas, while people with type 2 diabetes are insensitive to insulin. So in both cases, there is a high level of blood sugar.

The levels of blood glucose during fasting give us insight into how the cells respond to blood sugar. A high level of blood glucose is indicative of the body's ability to lower blood glucose, and the conclusion might be either high insulin resistance or insufficient insulin production. Prolonged fasting has the effect of minimizing blood glucose levels. The sugars in the blood get used up, albeit slowly.

There are two methods of testing the level of blood sugar: the traditional blood sugar test, and the glycosylated hemoglobin (HbAlc). The glycosylated hemoglobin test is for checking how blood glucose has been changing. The traditional method of checking blood sugar involves daily tests which may be conducted by the affected person.

Developing Your Fasting Regimen

There are some fasting regimens. All of them have their pros and cons. They are only as good as the person trying to follow them. During fasts, it is recommended to take water to flush out toxins and also to mitigate hunger. However, if you want to improve the success rate of your fast, you might consider dry fasts, where you don't consume any fluid.

You may perform a fast for as short a time as a couple of hours or as long as a full week (and maybe even more, depending on your stamina). However, if your goal is to lose weight, then shorter fasts are more effective. For instance, intermittent fasting is many times more fruitful than prolonged fasting, but ultimately, you get to choose what you feel will work for you.

Short fasts allow you to go through a cycle of fasting and eating windows. You start by creating a plan in which you detail your period of fasting and when your eating window opens. During the eating window, it is advisable to consume unprocessed foods and avoid sugar-laden foods. This will boost your insulin sensitivity.

Long fasts have their benefits too, but on the whole, they are much less rewarding than short fasts. The strain associated with long fasts make you susceptible to infections and might, in the worst case scenario, rewire your physiological functions.

Things to Incorporate to Make Fasting Safe for Diabetics

When a diabetic goes on a fast, their body secretes the glucagon hormone, which leads to a spike in the blood sugar level. Thus, a diabetic should start by informing themselves properly before they deprive themselves of food.

The first thing is to determine whether they are fit to fast. A diabetic person should seek medical clearance before they attempt fasting. A person with advanced diabetes will have a low blood sugar level. If they go on a fast, they risk falling into a coma. A medical professional offers the best counsel as to how to conduct the fast and for how long.

For type 1 diabetics, it is important to have a test kit to observe the fluctuation of blood sugar throughout the fast. This helps in tweaking the fast or deciding whether to call it off.

Another safety measure is to have a confidant know of their fasting. The psycho-social support offered by a confidant would keep them going. The confidant should be someone in their close proximity that can monitor their progress.

Diabetics should indulge in a balanced diet during their eating window. A balanced diet comprises of foods rich in minerals and vitamins. One common thing that fasting induces is cravings. Fast foods, for instance, are sugar-laden and they have no real nutritional value. Indulging in fast foods during eating windows only negates the effectiveness of the fast.

A diabetic should know when to quit and how to quit. If there is a massive fluctuation of blood glucose, or if a complication develops, then that's a hint to quit. Towards the end of the fast, a diabetic should consume light meals first, and then transition back to their normal eating patterns.

Role of Supplements

A supplement is a substance that enhances the food that a person eats. The common types of ingredients in supplements include vitamins, minerals, botanicals, amino acids, enzymes, organ tissues, and glandulars. The supplements are critical in optimizing nutritional value of food. The water-soluble ingredients of supplements are metabolized and eliminated from the body same day, while fat-soluble elements may be stored in the body for several days or even weeks. Supplements may be taken on either a daily basis or alternately—depending on the elements they provide to the body. One should always seek the guidance of a medical professional about the number of supplements to consume.

Supplements are not as critical during short fasts as they are in prolonged fasts. The body is a store of many nutritional elements, and fasting induces the body to tap into its reservoirs, but it is still important to take supplements to discourage nutrition deficiency. Fat-soluble vitamins need to be taken alongside fats to make for easy absorption. They include vitamin A, vitamin D, vitamin E, and vitamin K. They are kept in body cells too. Water-soluble vitamins are eliminated on the same day, especially if your body is well hydrated. Water-soluble vitamins include B3, B2, B1, and acids. If you have a poor diet, water-soluble vitamins are stable sources of nutrition.

The primary function of supplements is to improve the nutritional value of a person's diet by supplying vital elements that are not easily accessible. Taking supplements while on a fast helps mitigate the side effects of fasting such as headaches and cramps.

Types of Supplements that Stabilize Electrolytes

Sodium. The intake of Sodium is dependent upon your level of physical activity. Generally, if you engage in tougher physical exercises, you should take a high dose. Sodium is vital in eliminating cramps and various pains in the body.

Potassium. This supplement is vital for the optimal functioning of the heart. Potassium deficiency is normally accompanied by problems such as increased heartbeat and blood pressure. Potassium also helps in the flow of blood. A person with potassium deficiency is bound to experience exhaustion and constant lethargic feeling.

Magnesium. People who are lacking in this vital nutrient experience a range of problems like low energy, anxiety, insomnia, indigestion, muscle aches, poor heart health, and migraines. Magnesium supplements help your body absorb magnesium at a higher rate. Magnesium should be taken alongside food as opposed to plainly for maximum health benefit.

Zinc. This supplement is very crucial in improving the health of an individual. It regulates appetite, improves taste, promotes weight loss, minimizes hair loss, mitigates digestive problems, and cures chronic fatigue. Additionally, zinc improves nerve health and boosts testosterone. Zinc, too, should be consumed alongside other meals for maximum health benefits.

Calcium. This supplement helps in strengthening the musculoskeletal frame of an individual, heart health, and reduces the risk of developing ailments like cancer and diabetes. Calcium and magnesium should be taken at separate times to avoid stunted absorption rates.

Iodine. Iodine is crucial in improving thyroid health. The thyroid gland secretes hormones that play a vital role in the basal metabolic rate.

How to Keep Insulin Levels Low

This hormone produced by the pancreas facilitates the absorption of sugars into body cells. The insulin levels should be stable for optimum metabolism to take place. High levels of insulin might lead to serious complications like high blood pressure. Someone with a high blood glucose level needs to lower their blood sugar level, else they may suffer serious health complications. Here are some of the ways to keep insulin levels low.

Diet. Your diet will have a direct impact on your blood sugar levels.

Sugary, fat-laden foods will raise your blood glucose through the roof. On the other hand, a low-carb diet will help keep your blood glucose levels down.

Portion. There is a direct correlation between the portion of your food and your blood sugar levels. A giant portion of your favorite dish will lead to a surge in blood glucose. On the other hand, a small portion will keep your blood sugar stable. Bearing this in mind, you should aim to take small portions of food, as they minimize the fluctuation of blood glucose levels.

Exercise regularly. You can bring the high blood sugar levels down through exercise. When you exercise, your body powers your activities with the glucose in your blood. So exercises—and in particular, aerobics—can lead to low blood glucose levels.

Drink water constantly. Staying hydrated is also important in keeping the blood sugar level down. Water will flush out toxins and help streamline your metabolism.

Avoid alcohol. Alcohol not only lowers your inhibitions and makes you indulge in unhealthy foods like fries and roast meat, but it is also calorie-packed. If you aim to minimize your blood sugar, restrict your alcohol intake or drop it altogether.

What Causes Insulin Resistance?

Insulin is produced by the pancreas, and its work is to facilitate absorption of glucose into body cells. Insulin resistance is a condition where body cells are insensitive to insulin. For that reason, the rate of conversion of sugars into energy is affected. What are some of the causes of this condition?

Obesity. Most obese people have a ton of toxic elements stashed in their body. The combination of high blood sugar levels and toxic elements promote cellular inflammation. These cells naturally become insulin resistant.

Inactivity. Insulin resistance is common in people who hardly ever move their limbs. They don't perform any physical activity, so their energy requirement (output) is minimal. This creates some sort of "cell apathy" and promotes insulin resistance.

Sleep apnea. This is a sleep disorder characterized by faulty breathing. People who suffer from sleep apnea snore loudly and also feel tired after a night's sleep. Studies have shown a link between sleep apnea and development of insulin resistance in body cells.

High blood pressure. High blood pressure or hypertension is a degenerative medical issue where the blood pressure in blood vessels is more than 140/90 mmHg. Hypertension makes the heart's task of pumping out blood more difficult and may contribute to complications such as atherosclerosis, stroke, and kidney disease. Studies have shown a correlation between people with high blood pressure and the development of insulin resistance.

Smoking. The habit of smoking can give you many health complications. One of them is the risk of cancer development. Additionally, smoking seems to promote insulin resistance.

How Insulin Resistance Affects the Body

Insulin resistance makes it hard for the body cells to absorb sugars, which leads to high blood glucose levels. Some of the causes of insulin resistance include obesity, poor diet, sleep disorders, and sedentary lifestyle.

The American Diabetes Association (ADA) has stated that there is a 70% chance for people with insulin resistance to develop type 2 diabetes if they don't change their habits.

Insulin resistance may trigger the development of acanthosis nigricans, a skin condition in which dark spots cover parts of the body, especially the neck region.

Insulin resistance enhances weight gain, because it slows down base metabolism, causing a surge of blood sugar levels. Insulin carries off the excess blood sugar into fat stores, and thus, the person gains weight.

Insulin resistance promotes high blood pressure. The elevated blood glucose levels cause the heart to have to struggle with pumping more blood, causing high blood pressure.

Insulin resistance causes constant thirst and hunger pangs. Insulin resistance promotes the miscommunication between brain receptors and body cells. Thus, the brain activates the hunger hormone and makes the person eternally hungry. If not corrected, this leads to overeating and eventually chronic obesity.

Insulin resistance weakens the body. Insulin resistance leads to low energy output. And for that reason, the body doesn't have a lot of energy to use up, which makes the person feel (and look) weak.

Insulin resistance makes you urinate frequently; the condition affects the efficiency of physiological functions, and one of the results is a constant need to urinate.

Insulin resistance makes the body more susceptible to attack by diseases.

The Role of Amylin

Amylin is a protein hormone. It is produced by the pancreas alongside insulin. Amylin helps in glycemic control by promoting the slow emptying of the gastric and giving feelings of satisfaction. Amylin discourages the upsurge of blood glucose levels.

Amylin is part of the endocrine system, and it plays a critical role in glycemic control. The hormone is secreted by the pancreas, and its main function is to slow down the rate of appearance of nutritional elements in the plasma. It complements insulin.

Amylin and Insulin are secreted in a ratio of 1:100. Amylin delays gastric emptying and decreases the concentration of glucose in the plasma, whereas insulin facilitates absorption of sugars into cells. Diabetic people lack this hormone.

The amylin hormone can coalesce and create amyloid fibers, which may help in destroying diabetes. Amylin is secreted when there is the stimulus of nutrition in the blood. Unlike insulin, it is not purged in the liver but by renal metabolism.

Recent studies have shown the effect of amylin on the metabolism of glucose. In rats, amylin promoted insulin resistance.

Amylin slows down the food movement through the gut. As the food stays longer in the stomach, the rate of conversion of these foods to sugars will be slower.

Amylin also prevents the secretion of glucagon. Glucagon causes a surge in blood sugar level. Amylin prevents the inappropriate secretion of glucagon, which might cause a post-meal spike in blood sugar.

Amylin enhances the feeling of satiety. By reducing appetite, amylin ensures low blood glucose levels.

How Amylin Deficiency Affects Your Body

Amylin regulates the concentration of glucose in the blood by preventing the secretion of glucagon and slowing down the movement of food along the gut. People who suffer from diabetes have an amylin deficiency that causes excessive amounts of glucose to flow into the blood.

Increased insulin. A deficiency in amylin causes an extreme surge in blood glucose levels. To mitigate this spike, the pancreas secretes more insulin to help in the absorption of sugars into body cells. Increased levels of insulin in the blood might lead to complications.

Insulin resistance. Amylin deficiency eventually leads to high blood glucose levels. This might cause insulin resistance in body cells and, in worst case scenarios, it might trigger the immune system to attack the pancreas. High insulin levels in the blood might trigger memory loss and might even induce a coma.

Diabetes. Amylin deficiency leads to the overproduction of insulin, which, in the long run, impairs the pancreas. When the normal working of the pancreas is damaged, diabetes may develop.

Weight gain. Amylin deficiency promotes insulin resistance. When body cells become insensitive to insulin, there is less sugar converted into energy. So, the blood glucose level remains high. Insulin is responsible for carrying off these sugars to be stored as fats. Instead of these sugars being used as energy, they end up being stored as fat in the cells, which is the start of weight gain.

Headache. Thanks to insulin resistance, the body cells lack a reliable source of energy, which causes the body to switch to burning fats as an alternative energy source. One of the side effects of this process is normally headache and nausea.

The Insulin Resistance Diet

Insulin resistance causes slower absorption of sugars into body cells. This condition is rampant in obese people and diabetics. It is projected that the number of diabetics in the next 20 years will be over 320 million. This indicates a very worrying trend of diabetes. One of the things we can do to fight against diabetes is to improve our diet. Studies have shown that weight loss is a very effective means of minimizing insulin resistance. Here are the components of an insulin resistant diet:

Low carbs. Food high in carbs are responsible for blood sugar spikes. High levels of blood glucose promote insulin resistance. To ensure a stable blood glucose level, you should stick to low-carb foods.

Avoid sugary drinks. The American Diabetes Association advises against consumption of sugary drinks. These drinks with high sugar content include fruit juice, corn syrup, and other concentrates. Sugary drinks have a high sugar content, and they spike blood sugar levels. So, it'd be prudent to stay away from sugary drinks.

More fiber. Fiber is important in reducing the blood glucose levels. It improves the digestive health and improves blood circulation.

Healthy fats. Monounsaturated fats are very critical in improving heart health and regulating insulin levels.

Protein. Studies show that dietary protein is beneficial for people who suffer from diabetes. Regular consumption of protein is important for muscle growth and bone mass.

Size. Instead of taking large servings of a meal, opt for smaller portions of food, so that your post-meal blood glucose levels may be stable.

The Best Food for Diabetics

Diabetics don't have the luxury of eating any food they might want. For instance, sugar-laden foods and high-fat foods would spike their blood sugar levels and worsen the condition. They should instead stick to foods that are sources of minerals and vitamins. Foods like:

Fish. Fish is an important source of omega-3 fatty acids. These fatty acids are especially great for people with heart health complications and those who are at risk of stroke. Omega three fatty acids also protect your blood vessels, as well as reduce inflammation. Studies show that people who consume fish on the regular have better heart health than those who don't.

Greens. They are very nutritious and have low calories. Leafy greens like kale and spinach are excellent sources of minerals and vitamins. Leafy greens reduce inflammation markers, as well improve blood pressure. They are also high in antioxidants.

Eggs. The good old egg has been abused at the hands of intellectual conmen who have long said, albeit incorrectly, that eggs are bad. Eggs are excellent for reducing heart disease complications and also decreasing inflammation markers. Regular consumption of eggs improves cholesterol and blood glucose levels.

Chia seeds. They are high in fiber, and this fiber is critical in lowering blood glucose levels as well as in slowing down the rate of movement of food along the gut.

Nuts. Nuts are both tasty and healthy. They are great sources of fiber and are low in carbs. Regular consumption improves heart health and reduces inflammation and improves blood circulation.

Summary

Type 2 diabetes is a degenerative disease that impairs the ability of the pancreas to produce insulin. The hormone insulin is produced by the pancreas, and its main function is to regulate the conversion of glucose to energy. The risk of developing diabetes can be greatly minimized by taking the two steps: losing weight and having a balanced diet. The number of people with diabetes is at an all-time high, and people in both developed and poor countries are battling the disease. Symptoms of type 2 diabetes include tiredness, never-ending thirst, the constant urge to pee, irritability, weak immune system, and shivering. A carbohydrate metabolism test determines how blood sugar reacts to fasting. During a fast, blood sugar levels go up. Supplements are necessary for supplying important nutrients that may not be in the diet. The intake of supplements should be daily for optimum results. The important supplements include sodium, potassium, magnesium, zinc, calcium, and iodine. These are some of the measures to take to keep insulin levels low: have a strict diet, consume small portions, exercise regularly, and drink water constantly.

Chapter 12: Fasting For Heart Health

How Fasting Improves Your Heart's Health

Numerous studies have shown that fasting has a positive impact on heart health. Many people who have gone on a fast have reported feeling energetic and livelier afterward, which could be attributed to improved blood flow and general heart health. However, you need to fast consistently to achieve results.

Improves your heartbeat. When you go on a fast, your body is free from the digestion load, and so it channels that energy into optimizing your physiological functions. Your heart stands to gain from the optimized body functions, especially improving your heartbeat.

Improves blood pressure. Studies show that fasting has a positive impact on blood pressure. The rate of blood pressure is affected by factors like weight gain and obesity. But since fasting helps in weight loss, it has the extended advantage of lowering blood pressure, which improves the overall heart health.

Reduces cholesterol. Regularly fasting helps in lowering bad cholesterol. Also, controlled fasting increases the base metabolic rate.

Improved blood vessel health. Fasting is critical in improving the health of blood vessels. When blood vessels are subjected to high blood pressure, they slowly start to wear out, and might eventually burst up—which could be fatal, especially in the case of arteries. But fasting helps reduce blood pressure and bad cholesterol. The result is improved blood flow and overall heart health.

Autophagy. Regular dry fasts trigger the body to digest its weak and damaged cells in a process known as autophagy. Cell autophagy is very crucial because it helps eliminate old and damaged cells and creates room for new cells. With a new batch of cells to work with, the heart health is given a tremendous boost.

Summary

Fasting has been shown to improve the health of the heart. When you are fasting, your body reserves energy that would have gone into digestion for purposes of improving the heart health. It can execute its physiological functions much better. Fasting has also been shown to improve blood pressure. Fasting helps reduce obesity and reduces weight gain. This causes massive improvement in blood pressure. Fasting also plays a critical role in reducing cholesterol. Bad cholesterol increases the rate of developing heart disease. Also, controlled fasting increases the base metabolic rate. Fasting also improves the health of blood vessels. High blood pressure might cause blood vessels to wear out slowly, but fasting has a restorative effect on the blood vessels. Fasting also allows the body to digest its weak cells and make room for new and powerful body cells.

Chapter 13: The General Results of Fasting

Positive Effects of Fasting

You will get varied results depending on your preferred method of fasting, whether it's intermittent fasting, alternate-day, or prolonged fasting. These are some of the positive effects of fasting:

Weight loss. Fasting is an efficient way of losing weight. A study in 2015 showed that alternate fasting for a week resulted in weight loss of up to seven percent. When your body uses up the glucose in your blood, it now turns to the fat reserves to power its bodily functions. This helps in achieving weight loss.

Release of the human growth hormone. The human growth hormone promotes the growth of muscles and reduces obesity. Fasting triggers the secretion of the human growth hormone. This hormone is very crucial in building your body cells.

Improves insulin sensitivity. Low insulin sensitivity restricts the absorption of sugars into body cells. This might lead to complications such as chronic weight gain. Fasting leads to high insulin sensitivity that helps in absorption of sugars into body cells.

Normalizes ghrelin levels. Ghrelin is the hunger hormone which sends out hunger signals. Most obese people have abnormal ghrelin hormone levels that keep them in a perpetual state of hunger. Fasting, however, remedies this situation by normalizing ghrelin hormone levels, and thus you can receive accurate signals about hunger.

Lowers triglyceride levels. Depriving yourself of food for a set period of time has the effect of lowering bad cholesterol, and in the process, triglycerides are reduced.

Slows down aging. Many studies have shown the link between fasting and increased longevity in animals. Fasting allows the body to cleanse itself, promotes cell autophagy, and in the long run, lengthens lifespan.

Negative Effects of Fasting

As much as fasting is a practice with many benefits, admittedly there is a dark side too. These are some of the negative effects of fasting:

Strained body. A prolonged fast might put a big deal of a strain on your body. This may alter—albeit slightly—the normal processes of your body. A prolonged fast might slow down the effectiveness of your body as the body adapts to survive on too little energy.

Headaches. Headaches are common during fasts, especially at the start. The headache is normally a response of the brain to diminished blood glucose levels that force the body to switch to burning fats as a source of energy.

Low blood pressure. Fasting is a major cause of low blood pressure. Low blood pressure slows down the conversion of sugars into energy. This may lead to complications such as temporary blindness and, in extreme cases, can induce a coma.

Eating disorders. For someone who's too eager, it is easy to abuse fasting and turn it into an eating disorder. The main aim of fasting is to improve health, but starving yourself and having an eating disorder is anything but healthy. Some of the eating disorders that people who fast are at risk of developing include anorexia and bulimia.

Cravings. The hunger triggered by fasting might cause us to overcompensate. We may develop cravings for fast foods and other unhealthy foods. During our eating window, we may find ourselves consuming a lot of unhealthy foods, under the delusion that the fast will override that.

Summary

Weight loss is one of the main benefits of fasting. When you fast, your blood glucose is diminished, and this forces your body to turn to fats as an alternative source of energy. Fasting also promotes the production of the human growth hormone. This is the hormone responsible for muscle growth. Fasting also improves insulin sensitivity. Low insulin sensitivity impairs the body's ability to convert sugars into energy. Fasting also leads to high insulin sensitivity that helps in the absorption of sugars into body cells. Fasting also helps normalize ghrelin levels. The ghrelin hormone is known as the hunger hormone. Most obese people have abnormally high ghrelin levels that give incorrect hunger signals and make the obese person perpetually hungry. Fasting helps in correcting this problem, and the obese person starts to receive accurate signals. The negative effects of fasting include straining the body, headaches, low blood pressure, and eating disorders.

Chapter 14: Nutrition

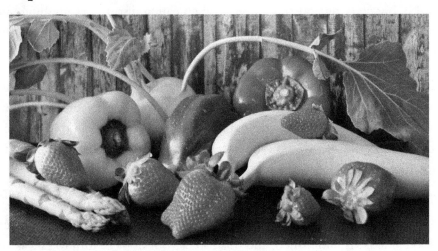

What Constitutes Good Nutrition?

Good nutrition implies a diet that contains all the required and important nutrients in appropriate proportions. When you fail to observe good nutrition, you risk developing complications from certain nutrient deficiencies. A good nutrition shouldn't be a one-off thing, but it should be a part of your lifestyle.

A great nutrition minimizes the risk of developing health complications such as diabetes, heart disease, and chronic weight gain. Here are the most important constituents of great nutrition:

- **Protein**

This nutrient is very important for muscle health, skin health, and hair. Also, it assists in the bodily reactions. Amino acids are essential for human growth and protein is stacked with amino acids. The best sources of protein include fish, eggs, and lentils.

- **Carbohydrates**

Carbohydrates are the main sources of energy for the body. They provide sugars that are converted into energy. There are two classes of carbohydrates: simple and complex. Simple carbohydrates are digested easily, and complex carbohydrates take time. Fruits and grains are some of the main sources of simple carbohydrates whereas beans and vegetables are sources of complex carbohydrates. For proper digestion, dietary fiber (carbohydrate) is needed. Men need a daily intake of 30 grams of fiber and women need 24 grams. Important sources of dietary fiber include legumes and whole grains.

- **Fats**

Fats play an essential role in health improvement. Both monounsaturated and polyunsaturated fats are healthy. Sources of monounsaturated fats include avocados and nuts. As for polyunsaturated fats, seafood is a major source. Unhealthy fats include trans fats and saturated fats, mostly found in junk food.

- **Vitamins**

Vitamins A, B, C, D, E, and K are necessary for the body's optimal functioning. A deficiency in the important vitamins can lead to serious health complications and weakened immune system.

- **Minerals**

Calcium, iron, zinc, and iodine are some of the essential minerals. They are found in a variety of foods including vegetables, grains, and meats.

- **Water**

Most of the human body is composed of water. It is a very essential nutrient for the proper functioning of the body.

Why Good Nutrition Is Important

The main reason why people ensure that they have a good nutrition is to improve their health. A good nutrition is essentially about consuming foods that are rich in vitamins, minerals, and fats. So, here are some of the reasons why good nutrition is vital.

Reduces risk of cancer. Good nutrition plays a vital role in optimizing your health. If you consume healthy food, you drastically reduce your chances of getting cancer, as many cancers are a result of bad lifestyle choices.

Reduces risk of developing high blood pressure. High blood pressure causes a strain on the heart. It also leads to the wearing and tearing of the blood vessels. Having good nutrition normalizes your blood pressure and thus improves your heart health.

Lowers cholesterol. Bad cholesterol leads to serious complications like heart disease. When you observe good nutrition that involves fruits and essential vitamins, the bad cholesterol is eliminated, thus improving the functioning of your body.

Increased energy. Bad food choices have a draining effect. However, nutritious foods replenish the body cells with vital nutrients, and thus the body is active. A nutritious diet is a key to improving productivity.

Improved immunity. Diseases are always looking for new victims. People who have a poor diet are bound to have a weak immune system. The weak immune system won't sufficiently protect them against attacks. On the other hand, people who consume a nutritious diet tend to have a strong immune system. This improved immunity keeps diseases at bay.

The Advantages of a High-Fat Diet

Many studies have shown that a low-carb, high-fat diet has many health benefits, including weight management, and reduced risk of diabetes, cancer, and Alzheimer's. A high-fat diet is characterized by low carbohydrate intake and high intake of fat. The low carbohydrate intake puts the body into ketosis, a condition that optimizes burning of fat and helps convert fat into ketone bodies that act as an energy source of the brain. These are some of the advantages of a high-fat diet:

Stronger immune system. Saturated fats are an ally of the immune system. They help fight off microbes, viruses, and fungi. Fats help in the fight against diseases. A great source of saturated fats includes butter and coconut.

Improves skin health and eyesight. When someone is lacking in fatty acids, they are likely to develop dry skin and eyes. Fatty acids help in improving skin elasticity and strengthening eyesight.

Lowers risk of heart disease. Saturated fats trigger production of good cholesterol, which is key in reducing the risk of heart disease. Saturated fats also help fight inflammation. A good source of saturated fats includes eggs and coconut oil.

Strong bones. Healthy fats improve the density of bones and thus minimize the risk of bone diseases. Fats promote healthy calcium metabolism. Fatty acids, too, play a critical role in minimizing the risk of bone complications such as osteoporosis.

Improves reproductive health. Fats play a critical role in the production of hormones that improve fertility in both men and women. A high-fat diet improves reproductive health and, in particular, the production of testosterone and estrogen.

Weight loss. A high-fat diet promotes high metabolism and, as a result, the body can crunch more calories, leading to weight loss.

Improved muscle gain. A high-fat diet promotes muscle gain. This is achieved through hormone production and speeding up cell recovery after strenuous exercise.

Role of Ketone Bodies

The three ketone bodies produced by the liver include acetoacetate, beta-hydroxybutyrate, and acetone. Ketone bodies are water-soluble, and it takes a blood or urine test to determine their levels.

Ketone bodies are oxidized in the mitochondria to provide energy. The heart uses fatty acids as fuel in normal circumstances, but during ketogenesis, it switches to ketone bodies. When the blood glucose levels are high, the body stores the excesses as fat. When you go for an extended period of time without eating, the blood glucose levels diminish. This triggers the body to convert fat into usable energy. Most body cells can utilize fatty acids, except the brain. The liver thus converts fats into ketone bodies and releases them into the blood to supply energy to the brain. When ketone bodies start to build up in the blood, problems might arise. An increase in the levels of acetone can induce acidosis, a condition where blood pH is lowered. Acidosis has a negative impact on most of the body cells, and in worst cases, it leads to death. With that in mind, it is prudent to replenish your body with carbohydrates as soon as ketosis kicks off. A person with type 1 diabetes is more susceptible to high levels of ketone bodies. For instance, when they fail to take an insulin shot, they will experience hypoglycemia. The combination of low blood glucose level and high glucagon level will cause the liver to produce ketone bodies at an alarming rate which might cause complications.

Benefits of the Ketogenic Diet

Here are some of the benefits associated with ketone bodies:

Treating Alzheimer's. Alzheimer's behaves in a way similar to diabetes. Essentially, it is the brain resisting insulin. Due to insulin resistance, the brain only gets minimal energy, which might cause the death of brain cells. However, ketone bodies are an alternative source of energy that the brain can utilize. Ketone bodies have been shown to prevent a buildup of compounds that enhance the development of Alzheimer.

Normalizes insulin production. Ketone bodies are only produced when blood glucose is low. For this reason, the pancreas stops pumping more insulin to aid in the absorption of sugars because the body has already switched into ketogenesis.

Regulates metabolism. Ketone bodies regulate metabolism through their effects on mitochondria. The mitochondria are the cells' power plants, and they respond better to energy from fats rather than glucose. In this sense, ketone bodies improve the functioning of the mitochondria.

Lowers hunger. When the body is utilizing ketone bodies, it seems that there's less of an urge to consume food. Ketogenesis regulates the hunger hormone. When a person is consuming fast foods, there is no end to the urge to take another serving. Eventually, this leads to weight gain.

Increases good cholesterol. The good cholesterol improves blood flow and the condition of your heart. Ketogenesis helps in the production of the good cholesterol and thus helps in improving heart health.

Improves brain health. Ketone bodies are especially effective as a source of energy for the brain. Many people who have practiced the ketone diet say that it improves their mental clarity and focus.

The Importance of a Well-Balanced Diet

When we talk about a balanced diet, we refer to a variety of foods that supply us with important nutrients such as protein, carbohydrates, healthy fats, vitamins, and minerals. So, what is the importance of a well-balanced diet?

Strengthens immune system. When you consume a diet that's rich in nutrients, your immune system will become stronger. This places your body in a far better place to fight disease vectors that might have otherwise overwhelmed your body's defense system.

Weight loss. In the past, obesity was a problem in only developed nations. Not anymore. Nowadays even poor people are struggling with obesity. This is partially due to fast foods being cheaper and more convenient. As you can imagine, obesity has become a crisis the world over. The open secret is that obesity can be mitigated through a balanced diet. A diet rich in nutritious elements will nourish your body and also regulate your appetite so that you don't fall into the temptation of eating unhealthy foods.

Mental health. People who observe a balanced diet are less likely to fall into bad moods and depression. The nutritious elements stabilize their emotions and enable them to be more resistant to the autosuggestions of their mind.

Skin health. Dry skin is often the result of a bad diet. When you have a balanced diet, your skin and hair are nourished, and it gives you a glow. Foods rich in vitamins and collagen improve skin elasticity.

Promotes growth. A balanced diet helps kids have a well-formed body as they transition into adults and it helps adults maintain a well-figured body.

Summary

A good nutrition is a diet that contains all the important nutrients in appropriate portions. You risk developing complications if you fail to follow a good nutrition. The risk of developing health complications is greatly minimized by a great nutrition. Protein is one of the most important elements of a good nutrition. It is important for muscle health, skin health and development of hair. Protein also plays a role in bodily reactions. Carbohydrates are the major source of energy. They provide glucose that the body cells use to power activities of the body. Fats also play an important role in improving health. Monounsaturated fats and polyunsaturated fats are especially healthy. Vitamins are necessary for the body to function optimally. Minerals and water are important too. People ensure that they have good nutrition to improve their health. They achieve this by consuming foods that are rich in nutritious elements. A high-fat diet promotes strong immunity, better eyesight, a lower risk of heart disease, and stronger bones.

Chapter 15: Exercise

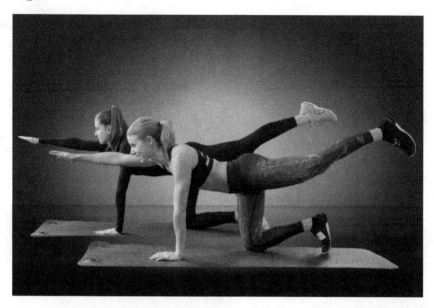

Pros of Exercising While Fasting

For the longest time, it was considered unhealthy to exercise while on a fast, but new evidence has shown that it is perfectly healthy to exercise even while you are fasting.

When you fast for health purposes, it shows that you are committed to improving your health and managing your weight. One of the ways you could get better results is by turning to physical exercise. A combination of intermittent fasting and physical exercise will burn up calories and help you reach your health goals in the shortest time possible.

The time of day that you exercise seems to affect the outcome. For instance, exercising in the morning right after you wake up promotes more weight loss than exercising at night. For intermittent fasting to be effective, you need to abstain from food for at least 16 hours.

When you exercise while on a fast, you speed up weight loss and optimize your health because of increased oxidation that promotes the growth of muscle cells.

It enriches your blood. Exercising has a positive effect on your breathing system and lung capacity. This helps in increasing the oxygen levels in your blood.

Exercising also improves heart health. Aerobic exercises, in particular, improve blood circulation and develop the stamina of the heart. Now, the blood pressure stabilizes and nutrients can spread to the whole body.

Exercising while on a fast improves your body's adaptability. It is never a good idea to idle around while on a fast, as it will trigger cravings. However, when you engage in physical activity, your body starts to adapt. It helps you create more stamina to endure your fast.

Best Exercises to Do

Exercising while fasting increases the rate of calorie burning. As a result, more weight is lost, and health is optimized in much less time. Here are the best exercises to perform while on a fast:

- **Aerobic exercise**

Aerobic exercise increases your heartbeat and breathing cycle. Aerobic exercise also improves lung capacity and heart health. Some of the benefits of aerobic exercise include improved mental health, minimized inflammation, lowered blood pressure, lowered blood sugar, and a minimized risk of heart disease, stroke, type 2 diabetes, and cancer. Aerobic exercises tend to be intense and easy to perform. Some examples of aerobic exercises include dancing, speed-walking, jogging, and cycling.

- **Strength training**

Strength training is important for muscle gain. People who perform strength training have more energy and keep their bodies at peak performance. Strength training improves your mental health, decreases blood sugar levels, enhances weight management, corrects posture, increases balance, and relieves pain in the back and joints. Strength training may be performed either in the gym or at home. Professional guidance depends on the exact exercise and equipment required. Strength training mostly takes the form of exercises such as pull-ups, push-ups, sit-ups, squats, and lunges. It is recommended to take breaks from strength training to allow muscle growth.

- **Stretching**

Stretching exercises are vital in improving the flexibility of a person. The exercises are designed to improve the strength and flexibility of tendons. Stretching exercises also improve the aesthetic quality of muscles. They also improve the circulation of blood and promote nourishment of all body cells.

- **Balance exercises**

Balance exercises promote agility. The exercises are designed to make your joints flexible. Balance exercises lead to improved focus and motor skills. The exercises include squats, sit-ups, and leg lifts.

Summary

Contrary to what people thought for the longest time, it is healthy to exercise while on a fast. A combination of exercise and fasting is a resource-intensive activity that makes your body burn more calories. Studies show that exercising in the morning has a far better outcome than exercising at night before bed. When you exercise while fasting, oxidation in cells promotes the growth of muscles. Exercising while on a fast also enriches your blood. The improved breathing cycle and lung capacity help in increasing the level of oxygen in the blood. Exercising is vital in improving heart health and blood circulation. It is never a good idea to stay idle while you are on a fast. Your hunger will be magnified, and it might cause to break the fast. Some of the best exercises to do for maximum weight loss and health improvement include aerobic exercises, strength training, stretching and balance exercises.

Chapter 16: Having a Partner to Keep You in Check

Role of a Partner

Depriving yourself of food is by no means easy. If you have no experience, the temptation to slide back is real. In some instances, fasting might make you lapse into a worse state than before. This is especially after a small duration of fasting where the hunger is extreme, and then you are tempted into eating unhealthy foods, trapping you into eating them.

Having a partner to keep you in check is a good step, and if they are into fasting themselves, that's even better. Ideally, your partner should be someone that "understands" you. He or she will make fasting less taxing. They will be there to see your progress and offer constructive criticism when needed. As your fasting progresses, they will help you adjust accordingly or make tweaks, to go through the fast in the safest manner possible.

Your partner will hold you accountable for your fasting journey. Attaining health goals is no easy task. It takes dedication, discipline, and consistency. It's exactly why you need a partner to hold you accountable when you stray or when you fall back on your goals. A responsible partner will be interested in your gains (i.e., asking questions about your weight loss so far and wanting to know what your diet is like).

A partner is also important because you have someone to talk to about your journey. They can offer you psychosocial support in your moments of vulnerability. It makes a world of difference. And you will stick to your goals knowing that someone cares.

Traits to Look for in a Partner

Not everyone may qualify to be a partner to someone who's fasting. The first thing to look out for is their opinion on the subject of fasting. Some people seem to think that fasting is a bad practice and a waste of time. Clearly, you wouldn't want such a person as your partner.

- **Patience**

Your partner should demonstrate patience. You cannot rush things while fasting. Sometimes, the results might take time, and in such situations, the last thing you want is someone on your neck, probably trashing your methods.

- **Observation skills**

A great partner must be a good observer. Their job is to spot loopholes that need to be closed, to assess situations, and to weigh overall progress. They need strong observation skills that will make them suitable for their positions. Also, remember that it is sometimes critical to call off a fast. Maybe you will be hard on yourself even when you are falling apart. An observant partner should notice the change and suggest that you stop.

- **Communication skills**

They should have good communication skills. What good is it to know something and not express it in a timely and appropriate fashion? A great partner should be very communicative and should express him/herself in an elaborate manner.

- **Knowledgeable**

A good partner should be knowledgeable. They should have a working knowledge of the whole subject of fasting. During every step of the fast, they should have a mental picture of what's coming. This will strengthen your bond and together you can meet any challenge.

- **Respect**

They should be able to respect you, your methods, and also have self-respect. This creates an enabling environment.

Should You Join A Support Group?
When your brain floods you with hunger hormones during a fast, the

temptation to quit is real. One of the methods to minimize your chances of quitting is to join a support group. This is ideally a group of people who have similar fasting pursuits as you. Now you have a family to keep you in check and boost your confidence.

A support network will allow you to cope and express your feelings and get connected with like-minded people. In times of vulnerability, others will come to your help. As other members share their experiences, you learn that you are not alone, and you even broaden your perspective and wisdom.

Support networks include people who are at various stages toward the common goal you all have. In times of conflict, you have ready help, and if you are at an advanced stage yourself, then you should offer help to those in need of it too. Support networks have non-judgmental environments and therapeutic effects.

The best support groups are those that foster frequent get-togethers. Ideally, the members should come from the same society, but that doesn't mean other kinds of support groups are necessary. For instance, you could join an online support network and be free to commune with your family at your convenience. Online support groups seem to be a thing nowadays. People from around the world with common goals are coming together to form support networks.

The most important thing when you join a support group is to become a giver rather than a taker. Or both. When everyone is interested in giving, you have a resourceful group of like-minded people.

Summary

People who are overwhelmed by the idea of staying without food should consider getting a partner. Your partner should help you cultivate a strong sense of discipline and stick to your routine. Ideally, your partner should be someone who understands you. He or she will help you get through fasting. A supportive partner is there to check your progress and offer constructive criticism when the occasion calls for it. He or she should be someone that you can open up to and express your fears and concerns. With the right partner, your fasting journey will be smooth and enjoyable. Your partner should be patient, observant, communicative, respectful, and knowledgeable. Joining a support group will help you come together with other like-minded people for a common goal. You are guaranteed of ready help and psychosocial support. The best support group to join should comprise of people from your local area, but it doesn't rule out joining even online support groups and communing with people from different parts of the world.

Chapter 17: Motivation

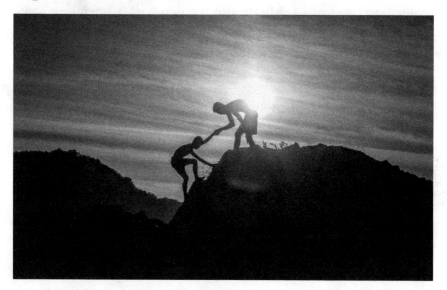

How to Stay Motivated Throughout Your Fast

Get a partner. If you go it alone, you are much more likely to forgive yourself and tweak the fast to suit you. For that reason, let there be a person to whom you are accountable. This person should put you in check and ensure that you follow the rules. Offer constructive criticism, and suggestions. A partner will help you stick to your routine. The ideal partner should be patient, empathetic, a good communicator, and knowledgeable about fasting. Let them share in your accomplishments as much as they have shared in your trials and struggle.

Seek knowledge. Being informed makes all the difference. You will know every possible outcome. You are aware of all the side effects of fasting and how to persist through the unpleasant experience instead of just quitting. Knowledge will help you optimize your fast and make you reap more benefits than anyone who had just deprived themselves of food. Being knowledgeable is important also in the sense that you are more aware of when to stop.

Set goals. Don't get into fasting with mental blindness. Instead, make an effort to set milestones. When you achieve a goal—for instance, when you hit your target weight—celebrate and then go back to reducing weight. Your brain responds to victory by making you feel confident. Now, you will have more confidence in your capacity to withstand hunger.

Develop positivity. A positive attitude makes all the difference. Keep reading about successful people who have achieved what you are looking for. Lockout all the negative energies that would derail you.

Record your progress. It is easy to underestimate yourself. As long as you keep going, the achievements will always be there. It's just a matter of recognizing them and celebrating.

How to Make Fasting Your Lifestyle
There are different approaches to fasting. You may fast every other day, once a week, or even a couple of times every month. In each instance, there are benefits.

But if you'd like to reap great benefits out of fasting, you should purposefully make it a daily ritual. Many people in the world today fast on a daily basis and have reported an increased quality of life.

The most common and most rewarding method is the 16:8 intermittent fasting. In this method, you fast for 16 hours in a day and then eat during the other 8 hours to complete the cycle.

Ideally, when you wake up, you should take a drink of water or black coffee and either exercise or just go on about your work. At around noon, your eating window opens, and you're free to have your meals up until 8 pm when the eating window closes.

During this eight-hour eating window, it is common to be tempted to overeat or indulge in unhealthy foods, thinking that the coming fast will "take care of that." Well, you must be careful not to fall into this temptation, or else your gains will be negated. Consume healthy and nutritious foods during the eating window and adhere to your 16-hour fast. The weight loss starts occurring in as short a span as a few days.

If you incorporate intermittent fasting into your lifestyle, the weight loss keeps going until you hit a stable weight where it plateaus. When fasting is your lifestyle, it makes your health improvement and weight loss permanent.

Summary

You need to take a few measures to stay motivated throughout the fast. One of the measures is to get a partner. A partner should hold you accountable and keep you in check so that you don't stray from the fasting routine. The ideal partner should be patient, empathetic, and a good communicator. Another way of motivating yourself is through seeking knowledge. As a knowledgeable person, you will be aware of all the responses that your body will give off. Knowledge will also help you optimize your fast and get the best possible results. Other ways to stay motivated throughout the fast include setting goals, developing positivity and recording your progress. If you make fasting part of your lifestyle, you stand to reap more benefits. The most common and most efficient fasting method is the 16:8, where you fast for 16 hours and then have an eating window of 8 hours.

Chapter 18: Foods for the Fast

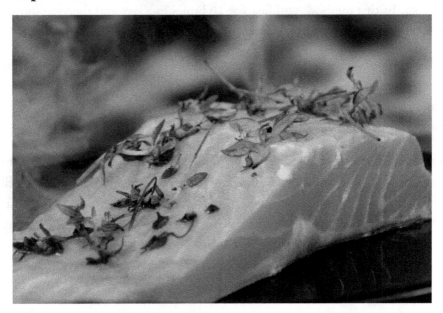

How Food Controls the Rate of the Success of Fasting

Depriving yourself of food is no easy task. Your body will tune up the hunger, and you will have to suppress the urge to feed. Not easy.

When you consume food, it is digested and released into the bloodstream as sugars. The pancreas secretes the hormone insulin to help in absorption of these sugars into body cells. When you stay for long without eating, there is no more food getting digested, and thus no more sugars getting released into the blood. The body soon runs out of the existing sugars and meets a crisis. The body is forced to switch to fats to provide energy for various physiological functions.

The foods that you eat have a massive impact on the efficacy of the fast. If you take light meals or small portions of food during the eating window, you will experience a higher degree of hunger during the fast. On the other side, if you consume large amounts of food during your eating window, your hunger will not be as intense.

One of the tricks to reducing hunger during the fast is to consume foods that are high in dietary fiber. Such foods make you full for a long time and will thus minimize the unpleasant feeling triggered by hunger.

Consuming healthy foods during your eating window is important. Some people fall into the temptation of eating unhealthy foods or even eating too much, and the effect is negative.

Intermittent fasting is favored by many people because it doesn't restrict consumption of foods, unlike fad diets that insist on vegan meals or raw food.

The Worst Foods to Take During Fasting

If you want to speed up your weight loss and avoid lifestyle diseases, these are some of the foods to cut back on, or maybe stay away from:

Sugary drinks. The high dose of fructose in sugary drinks will cause an extreme surge of blood sugar levels. High amounts of this kind of sugar promote insulin resistance and liver disease. High levels of insulin resistance have a negative impact on the absorption of sugars into body cells. This creates the perfect recipe for the development of heart disease and diabetes.

Junk food. They might taste heavenly, but the ingredients of most junk foods come from hell. Junk foods have almost zero nutritional value. Fries are prepared using hydrogenated oil that contains trans fats. Studies have been made on trans fats, and the conclusion is that continued consumption of trans fats leads to heart complications and cancer.

Processed food. Most processed foods have a long shelf life thanks to a host of nasty chemicals poured into them. The processed foods are made durable to gain a commercial edge over organic products with a limited shelf life. Most processed foods are high in sugars, sodium, and have low fiber content and nutrients.

White bread and cakes. Baked goods tend to affect people with celiac disease, most especially. But more than that, most of these baked goods are stashed with processed ingredients—sugars and fats—and they are low on fiber. Most baked goods trigger abnormal surges in blood sugar levels and increase the risk of heart disease.

Alcohol. Studies show that alcohol induces inflammation on the liver. Excessive alcohol consumption will eliminate all the successes of your fast and promote weight gain and even development of diabetes.

Seed oils. Studies show that these oils are unnatural. They contain harmful fatty acids that increase the risk of developing heart complications.

The Best Foods to Take During Fasting

These are some of the best foods to indulge in while you fast to reach your important health goals:

Nuts. Nuts are rich in nutritional value. Almonds, Brazil nuts, lentils, oatmeal, etc. have properties that help in the production of good cholesterol. Good cholesterol promotes heart health. Nuts are excellent sources of vitamins and minerals. Oatmeal, in particular, is essential in normalizing blood glucose levels.

Fruits and greens. They are important sources of essential nutrients that improve both gut health and brain health. Broccoli is rich in phytonutrients that reduce the risk of heart complications and cancers. Apples contain antioxidants that eliminate harmful radicals. Kale contains the vital vitamin K. Blueberries are excellent sources of fiber and phytonutrients. Avocados are good sources of monounsaturated fats that lower bad cholesterol and improve heart health.

White meats. These are an excellent source of protein and fatty acids. Fish provide omega-3 fatty acids which improve heart health and stimulate muscle growth. Chicken is a great source of protein, and it promotes the growth of muscle cells.

Grains. They are excellent sources of protein and dietary fiber that will keep you full. Grains also help in improving heart health and normalizing blood pressure.

Eggs. Eggs are excellent sources of protein, and they tend to fill you up thus minimizing hunger levels.

Tubers. Foods such as potatoes and sweet potatoes are loaded with essential vitamins and carbohydrates.

Dairy. Dairy seems to reduce the risk of development of obesity and type 2 diabetes. Cheese and whole milk are excellent sources of protein and essential minerals that promote bone development.

Summary

When you go on a fast, your body increases the hunger levels in an attempt to pressure you to look for food. Staying without food for a long time causes the body to switch to fats as an alternative energy source. When the carbohydrates supplying energy to the brain are depleted, the liver produces ketone bodies to supply energy to the brain. The food you eat (and the portion) will impact your hunger levels during the fast. It is important to consume healthy foods during the eating window no matter how strong the temptation to stray is. Some of the worst foods that you can indulge in while fasting includes sugary drinks, junk foods, processed foods, white bread and cakes, alcohol, and seed oils. On the other hand, some of the best foods you can indulge in would be nuts, fruits and greens, white meat, grains, eggs, tubes, and dairy.

PART III

Smoothie Diet Recipes

The smoothie diet is all about replacing some of your meals with smoothies that are loaded with veggies and fruits. It has been found that the smoothie diet is very helpful in losing weight along with excess fat. The ingredients of the smoothies will vary, but they will focus mainly on vegetables and fruits. The best part about the smoothie diet is that there is no need to count your calorie intake and less food tracking. The diet is very low in calories and is also loaded with phytonutrients.

Apart from weight loss, there are various other benefits of the smoothie diet. It can help you to stay full for a longer time as most smoothies are rich in fiber. It can also help you to control your cravings as smoothies are full of flavor and nutrients. Whenever you feel like snacking, just prepare a smoothie, and you are good to go. Also, smoothies can aid in digestion as they are rich in important minerals and vitamins. Fruits such as mango are rich in carotenoids that can help in improving your skin quality. As the smoothie diet is mainly based on veggies and fruits, it can detoxify your body.

In this section, you will find various recipes of smoothies that you can include in your smoothie diet.

Chapter 1: Fruit Smoothies

The best way of having fruits is by making smoothies. Fruit smoothies can help you start your day with loads of nutrients so that you can remain energetic throughout the day. Here are some easy-to-make fruit smoothie recipes that you can enjoy during any time of the day.

Quick Fruit Smoothie

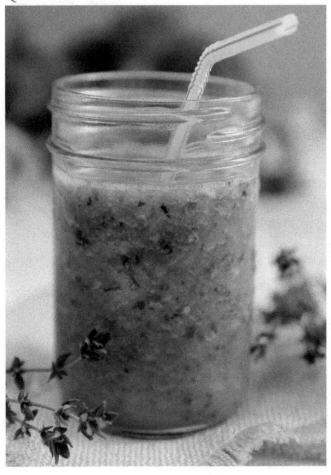

Total Prep & Cooking Time: Fifteen minutes

Yields: Four servings

Nutrition Facts: Calories: 115.2 | Protein: 1.2g | Carbs: 27.2g | Fat: 0.5g | Fiber: 3.6g

Ingredients

- One cup of strawberries
- One banana (cut in chunks)
- Two peaches
- Two cups of ice
- One cup of orange and mango juice

Method:

1. Add banana, strawberries, and peaches in a blender.

2. Blend until frothy and smooth.

3. Add the orange and mango juice and blend again. Add ice for adjusting the consistency and blend for two minutes.

4. Divide the smoothie in glasses and serve with mango chunks from the top.

Triple Threat Smoothie
Total Prep & Cooking Time: Ten minutes

Yields: Four servings

Nutrition Facts: Calories: 132.2 | Protein: 3.4g | Carbs: 27.6g | Fat: 1.3g | Fiber: 2.7g

Ingredients

- One kiwi (sliced)
- One banana (chopped)
- One cup of each
  - Ice cubes
  - Strawberries
- Half cup of blueberries
- One-third cup of orange juice
- Eight ounces of peach yogurt

Method:

1. Add kiwi, strawberries, and bananas in a food processor.

2. Blend until smooth.

3. Add the blueberries along with orange juice. Blend again for two minutes.

4. Add peach yogurt and ice cubes. Give it a pulse.

5. Pour the prepared smoothie in smoothie glasses and serve with blueberry chunks from the top.

Tropical Smoothie

Total Prep & Cooking Time: Fifteen minutes

Yields: Two servings

Nutrition Facts: Calories: 127.3 | Protein: 1.6g | Carbs: 30.5g | Fat: 0.7g | Fiber: 4.2g

Ingredients

- One mango (seeded)
- One papaya (cubed)
- Half cup of strawberries
- One-third cup of orange juice
- Five ice cubes

Method:

1. Add mango, strawberries, and papaya in a blender. Blend the ingredients until smooth.

2. Add ice cubes and orange juice for adjusting the consistency.

3. Blend again.

4. Serve with strawberry chunks from the top.

Fruit and Mint Smoothie

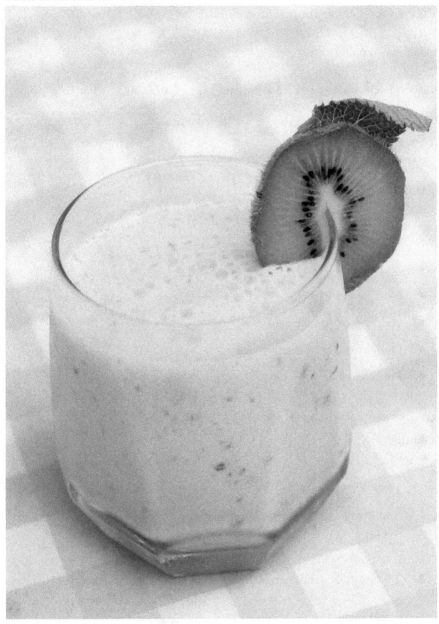

Total Prep & Cooking Time: Fifteen minutes

Yields: Two servings

Nutrition Facts: Calories: 90.3 | Protein: 0.7g | Carbs: 21.4g | Fat: 0.4g | Fiber: 2.5g

Ingredients

- One-fourth cup of each
  - Applesauce (unsweetened)
  - Red grapes (seedless, frozen)
- One tbsp. of lime juice
- Three strawberries (frozen)
- One cup of pineapple cubes
- Three mint leaves

Method:

1. Add grapes, lime juice, and applesauce in a blender. Blend the ingredients until frothy and smooth.

2. Add pineapple cubes, mint leaves, and frozen strawberries in the blender. Pulse the ingredients for a few times until the pineapple and strawberries are crushed.

3. Serve with mint leaves from the top.

Banana Smoothie

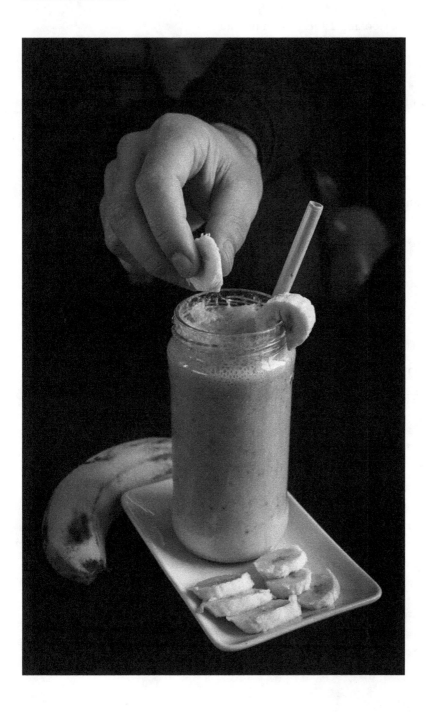

Total Prep & Cooking Time: Ten minutes

Yields: Four servings

Nutrition Facts: Calories: 122.6 | Protein: 1.3g | Carbs: 34.6g | Fat: 0.4g | Fiber: 2.2g

Ingredients

- Three bananas (sliced)
- One cup of fresh pineapple juice
- One tbsp. of honey
- Eight cubes of ice

Method:

1. Combine the bananas and pineapple juice in a blender.

2. Blend until smooth.

3. Add ice cubes along with honey.

4. Blend for two minutes.

5. Serve immediately.

Dragon Fruit Smoothie

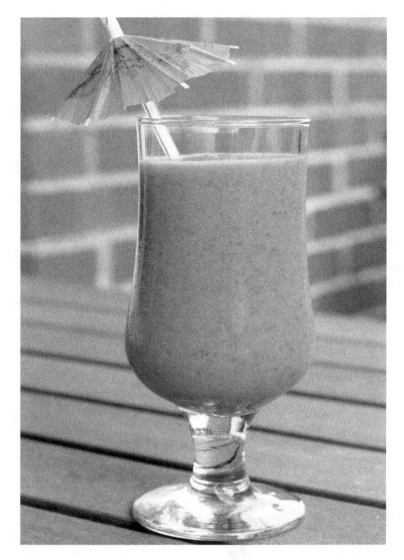

Total Prep & Cooking Time: Twenty minutes

Yields: Four servings

Nutrition Facts: Calories: 147.6 | Protein: 5.2g | Carbs: 21.4g | Fat: 6.4g | Fiber: 2.9g

Ingredients

- One-fourth cup of almonds
- Two tbsps. of shredded coconut
- One tsp. of chocolate chips
- One cup of yogurt
- One dragon fruit (chopped)
- Half cup of pineapple cubes
- One tbsp. of honey

Method:

1. Add almonds, dragon fruit, coconut, and chocolate chips in a high power blender. Blend until smooth.

2. Add yogurt, pineapple, and honey. Blend well.

3. Serve with chunks of dragon fruit from the top.

Kefir Blueberry Smoothie

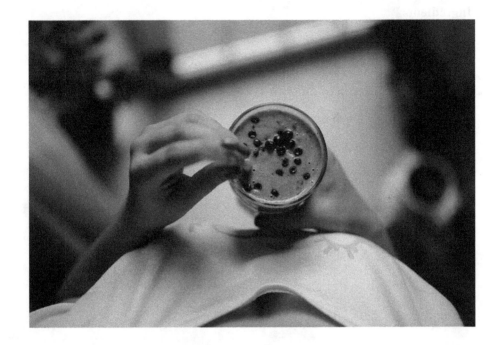

Total Prep & Cooking Time: Fifteen minutes

Yields: Two servings

Nutrition Facts: Calories: 304.2 | Protein: 7.3g | Carbs: 41.3g | Fat: 13.2g | Fiber: 4.6g

Ingredients

- Half cup of kefir
- One cup of blueberries (frozen)
- Half banana (cubed)

- One tbsp. of almond butter
- Two tsps. of honey

Method:

1. Add blueberries, banana cubes, and kefir in a blender.

2. Blend until smooth.

3. Add honey and almond butter.

4. Pulse the smoothie for a few times.

5. Serve immediately.

Ginger Fruit Smoothie

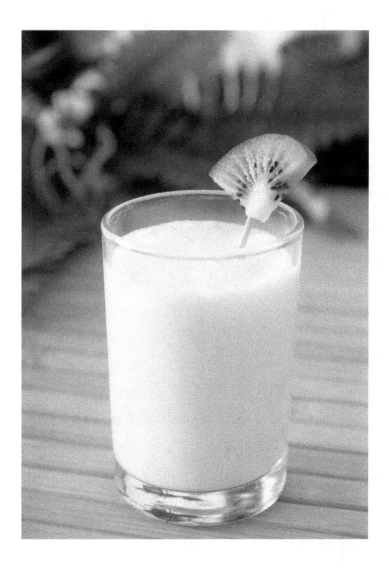

Total Prep & Cooking Time: Fifteen minutes

Yields: Two servings

Nutrition Facts: Calories: 160.2 | Protein: 1.9g | Carbs: 41.3g | Fat: 0.7g | Fiber: 5.6g

Ingredients

- One-fourth cup of each
    - Blueberries (frozen)
    - Green grapes (seedless)
- Half cup of green apple (chopped)
- One cup of water
- Three strawberries
- One piece of ginger
- One tbsp. of agave nectar

Method:

1. Add blueberries, grapes, and water in a blender. Blend the ingredients.

2. Add green apple, strawberries, agave nectar, and ginger. Blend for making thick slushy.

3. Serve immediately.

Fruit Batido

Total Prep & Cooking Time: Fifteen minutes

Yields: Six servings

Nutrition Facts: Calories: 129.3 | Protein: 4.2g | Carbs: 17.6g | Fat: 4.6g | Fiber: 0.6g

Ingredients

- One can of evaporated milk
- One cup of papaya (chopped)
- One-fourth cup of white sugar
- One tsp. of vanilla extract
- One tsp. of cinnamon (ground)
- One tray of ice cubes

Method:

1. Add papaya, white sugar, cinnamon, and vanilla extract in a food processor. Blend the ingredients until smooth.

2. Add milk and ice cubes. Blend for making slushy.

3. Serve immediately.

Banana Peanut Butter Smoothie
Total Prep & Cooking Time: Ten minutes

Yields: Four servings

Nutrition Facts: Calories: 332 | Protein: 13.2g | Carbs: 35.3g | Fat: 17.8g | Fiber: 3.9g

Ingredients

- Two bananas (cubed)
- Two cups of milk
- Half cup of peanut butter
- Two tbsps. of honey
- Two cups of ice cubes

Method:

1. Add banana cubes and peanut butter in a blender. Blend for making a smooth paste.

2. Add milk, ice cubes, and honey. Blend the ingredients until smooth.

3. Serve with banana chunks from the top.

Chapter 2: Breakfast Smoothies

Smoothie forms an essential part of breakfast in the smoothie diet plan. Here are some breakfast smoothie recipes for you that can be included in your daily breakfast plan.

Berry Banana Smoothie
Total Prep & Cooking Time: Twenty minutes

Yields: Two servings

Nutrition Facts: Calories: 330 | Protein: 6.7g | Carbs: 56.3g | Fat: 13.2g | Fiber: 5.5g

Ingredients

- One cup of each
  - Strawberries
  - Peaches (cubed)
  - Apples (cubed)
- One banana (cubed)
- Two cups of vanilla ice cream
- Half cup of ice cubes
- One-third cup of milk

Method:

1. Place strawberries, peaches, banana, and apples in a blender. Pulse the ingredients.

2. Add milk, ice cream, and ice cubes. Blend the smoothie until frothy and smooth.

3. Serve with a scoop of ice cream from the top.

Berry Surprise

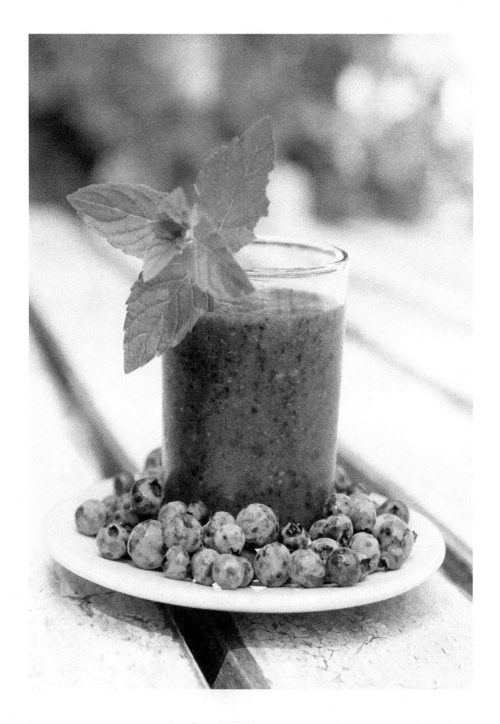

Total Prep & Cooking Time: Ten minutes

Yields: Two servings

Nutrition Facts: Calories: 164.2 | Protein: 1.2g | Carbs: 40.2g | Fat: 0.4g | Fiber: 4.8g

Ingredients

- One cup of strawberries
- Half cup of pineapple cubes
- One-third cup of raspberries
- Two tbsps. of limeade concentrate (frozen)

Method:

1. Combine pineapple cubes, strawberries, and raspberries in a food processor. Blend the ingredients until smooth.

2. Add the frozen limeade and blend again.

3. Divide the smoothie in glasses and serve immediately.

Coconut Matcha Smoothie

Total Prep & Cooking Time: Twenty minutes

Yields: Two servings

Nutrition Facts: Calories: 362 | Protein: 7.2g | Carbs: 70.1g | Fat: 8.7g | Fiber: 12.1g

Ingredients

- One large banana
- One cup of frozen mango cubes
- Two leaves of kale (torn)
- Three tbsps. of white beans (drained)
- Two tbsps. of shredded coconut (unsweetened)
- Half tsp. of matcha green tea (powder)
- Half cup of water

Method:

1. Add cubes of mango, banana, white beans, and kale in a blender. Blend all the ingredients until frothy and smooth.

2. Add shredded coconut, white beans, water, and green tea powder. Blend for thirty seconds.

3. Serve with shredded coconut from the top.

Cantaloupe Frenzy

Total Prep & Cooking Time: Ten minutes

Yields: Three servings

Nutrition Facts: Calories: 108.3 | Protein: 1.6g | Carbs: 26.2g | Fat: 0.2g | Fiber: 1.6g

Ingredients

- One cantaloupe (seeded, chopped)
- Three tbsps. of white sugar
- Two cups of ice cubes

Method:

1. Place the chopped cantaloupe along with white sugar in a blender. Puree the mixture.

2. Add cubes of ice and blend again.

3. Pour the smoothie in serving glasses. Serve immediately.

Berry Lemon Smoothie

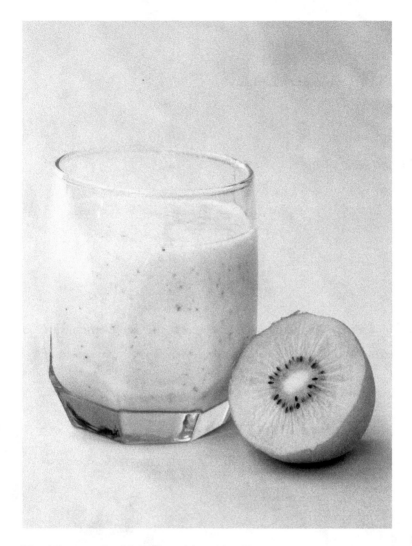

Total Prep & Cooking Time: Ten minutes

Yields: Four servings

Nutrition Facts: Calories: 97.2 | Protein: 5.4g | Carbs: 19.4g | Fat: 0.4g | Fiber: 1.8g

Ingredients

- Eight ounces of blueberry yogurt
- One and a half cup of milk (skim)
- One cup of ice cubes
- Half cup of blueberries
- One-third cup of strawberries
- One tsp. of lemonade mix

Method:

1. Add blueberry yogurt, skim milk, blueberries, and strawberries in a food processor. Blend the ingredients until smooth.

2. Add lemonade mix and ice cubes. Pulse the mixture for making a creamy and smooth smoothie.

3. Divide the smoothie in glasses and serve.

Orange Glorious

Total Prep & Cooking Time: Ten minutes

Yields: Four servings

Nutrition Facts: Calories: 212 | Protein: 3.4g | Carbs: 47.3g | Fat: 1.5g | Fiber: 0.5g

Ingredients

- Six ounces of orange juice concentrate (frozen)
- One cup of each
    - Water
    - Milk
- Half cup of white sugar
- Twelve ice cubes
- One tsp. of vanilla extract

Method:

1. Combine orange juice concentrate, white sugar, milk, and water in a blender.

2. Add vanilla extract and ice cubes. Blend the mixture until smooth.

3. Pour the smoothie in glasses and enjoy!

Grapefruit Smoothie

Total Prep & Cooking Time: Ten minutes

Yields: Two servings

Nutrition Facts: Calories: 200.3 | Protein: 4.7g | Carbs: 46.3g | Fat: 1.2g | Fiber: 7.6g

Ingredients

- Three grapefruits (peeled)
- One cup of water
- Three ounces of spinach
- Six ice cubes
- Half-inch piece of ginger
- One tsp. of flax seeds

Method:

1. Combine spinach, grapefruit, and ginger in a high power blender. Blend until smooth.

2. Add water, flax seeds, and ice cubes. Blend smooth.

3. Pour the smoothie in glasses and serve.

Sour Smoothie

Total Prep & Cooking Time: Ten minutes

Yields: Two servings

Nutrition Facts: Calories: 102.6 | Protein: 2.3g | Carbs: 30.2g | Fat: 0.7g | Fiber: 7.9g

Ingredients

- One cup of ice cubes
- Two fruit limes (peeled)
- One orange (peeled)
- One lemon (peeled)
- One kiwi (peeled)
- One tsp. of honey

Method:

1. Add fruit limes, lemon, orange, and kiwi in a food processor. Blend until frothy and smooth.

2. Add cubes of ice and honey. Pulse the ingredients.

3. Divide the smoothie in glasses and enjoy!

Ginger Orange Smoothie
Total Prep & Cooking Time: Ten minutes

Yields: One serving

Nutrition Facts: Calories: 115.6 | Protein: 2.2g | Carbs: 27.6g | Fat: 1.3g | Fiber: 5.7g

Ingredients

- One large orange
- Two carrots (peeled, cut in chunks)
- Half cup of each
  - Red grapes
  - Ice cubes
- One-fourth cup of water
- One-inch piece of ginger

Method:

1. Combine carrots, grapes, and orange in a high power blender. Blend until frothy and smooth.

2. Add ice cubes, ginger, and water. Blend the ingredients for thirty seconds.

3. Serve immediately.

Cranberry Smoothie

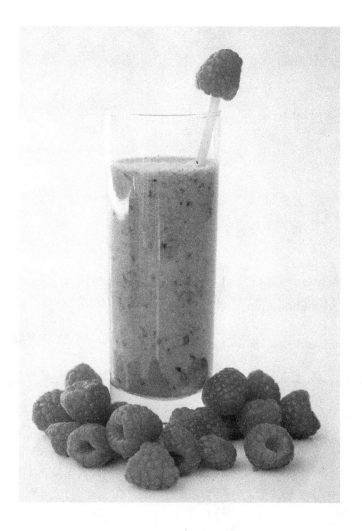

Total Prep & Cooking Time: One hour and ten minutes

Yields: Two servings

Nutrition Facts: Calories: 155.9 | Protein: 2.2g | Carbs: 33.8g | Fat: 1.6g | Fiber: 5.2g

Ingredients

- One cup of almond milk
- Half cup of mixed berries (frozen)
- One-third cup of cranberries
- One banana

Method:

1. Blend mixed berries, banana, and cranberries in a high power food processor. Blend until smooth.

2. Add almond milk and blend again for twenty seconds.

3. Refrigerate the prepared smoothie for one hour.

4. Serve chilled.

Creamsicle Smoothie

Total Prep & Cooking Time: Ten minutes

Yields: Two servings

Nutrition Facts: Calories: 121.3 | Protein: 4.7g | Carbs: 19.8g | Fat: 2.5g | Fiber: 0.3g

Ingredients

- One cup of orange juice
- One and a half cup of crushed ice
- Half cup of milk
- One tsp. of white sugar

Method:

1. Blend milk, orange juice, white sugar, and ice in a high power blender.

2. Keep blending until there is no large chunk of ice. Try to keep the consistency of slushy.

3. Serve immediately.

Sunshine Smoothie

Total Prep & Cooking Time: Thirty minutes

Yields: Four servings

Nutrition Facts: Calories: 176.8 | Protein: 4.2g | Carbs: 39.9g | Fat: 1.3g | Fiber: 3.9g

Ingredients

- Two nectarines (pitted, quartered)
- One banana (cut in chunks)
- One orange (peeled, quartered)
- One cup of vanilla yogurt
- One-third cup of orange juice
- One tbsp. of honey

Method:

1. Add banana chunks, nectarines, and orange in a blender. Blender for two minutes.

2. Add vanilla yogurt, honey, and orange juice. Blend the ingredients until frothy and smooth.

3. Pour the smoothie in glasses and serve.

- Two carrots

- Two cups of coconut milk (light)

- One small beet (quartered)

Method:

1. Add strawberries, raspberries, and orange in a blender. Blend until frothy and smooth.

2. Add beet, carrots, and coconut milk.

3. Blend again for one minute.

4. Divide the smoothie in glasses and serve.

Butternut Squash Smoothie

Total Prep & Cooking Time: Five minutes

Yields: Four servings

Nutrition Facts: Calories: 127.3 | Protein: 2.3g | Carbs: 32.1g | Fat: 1.2g | Fiber: 0.6g

Ingredients

- Two cups of almond milk
- One-fourth cup of nut butter (of your choice)
- One cup of water
- One and a half cup of butternut squash (frozen)
- Two ripe bananas
- One tsp. of cinnamon (ground)
- Two tbsps. of hemp protein
- Half cup of strawberries
- One tbsp. of chia seeds
- Half tbsp. of bee pollen

Method:

1. Add butternut squash, bananas, strawberries, and almond milk in a blender. Blend until frothy and smooth.

2. Add water, nut butter, cinnamon, hemp protein, chia seeds, and bee pollen. Blend the ingredients f0r two minutes.

3. Divide the smoothie in glasses and enjoy!

Zucchini and Wild Blueberry Smoothie

Total Prep & Cooking Time: Ten minutes

Yields: Three servings

Nutrition Facts: Calories: 190.2 | Protein: 7.3g | Carbs: 27.6g | Fat: 8.1g | Fiber: 5.7g

Ingredients

- One banana
- One cup of wild blueberries (frozen)
- One-fourth cup of peas (frozen)
- Half cup of zucchini (frozen, chopped)
- One tbsp. of each
  - Hemp hearts
  - Chia seeds
  - Bee pollen
- One-third cup of almond milk
- Two tbsps. of nut butter (of your choice)
- Ten cubes of ice

Method:

1. Add blueberries, banana, peas, and zucchini in a high power blender. Blend the ingredients for two minutes.

2. Add chia seeds, hemp hearts, almond milk, bee pollen, nut butter, and ice. Blend the mixture for making a thick and smooth smoothie.

3. Pour the smoothie in glasses and serve with chopped blueberries from the top.

Cauliflower and Blueberry Smoothie

Total Prep & Cooking Time: Five minutes

Yields: Two servings

Nutrition Facts: Calories: 201.9 | Protein: 7.1g | Carbs: 32.9g | Fat: 10.3g | Fiber: 4.6g

Ingredients

- One Clementine (peeled)
- Three-fourth cup of cauliflower (frozen)
- Half cup of wild blueberries (frozen)
- One cup of Greek yogurt
- One tbsp. of peanut butter
- Bunch of spinach

Method:

1. Add cauliflower, Clementine, and blueberries in a blender. Blend for one minute.

2. Add peanut butter, spinach, and yogurt. Pulse the ingredients for two minutes until smooth.

3. Divide the prepared smoothie in glasses and enjoy!

Immunity Booster Smoothie

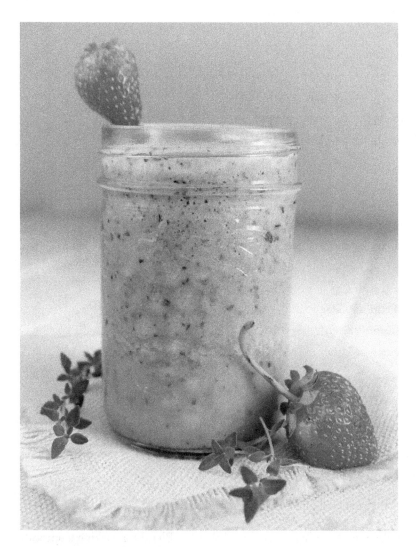

Total Prep & Cooking Time: Ten minutes

Yields: Two servings

Nutrition Facts: Calories: 301.9 | Protein: 5.4g | Carbs: 70.7g | Fat: 4.3g | Fiber: 8.9g

Ingredients

For the orange layer:

- One persimmon (quartered)
- One ripe mango (chopped)
- One lime (juiced)
- One tbsp. of nut butter (of your choice)
- Half tsp. of turmeric powder
- One pinch of cayenne pepper
- One cup of coconut milk

For the pink layer:

- One small beet (cubed)
- One cup of berries (frozen)
- One pink grapefruit (quartered)
- One-fourth cup of pomegranate juice
- Half cup of water
- Six leaves of mint
- One tsp. of honey

Method:

1. Add the ingredients for the orange layer in a blender. Blend for making a smooth liquid.

2. Pour the orange liquid evenly in serving glasses.

3. Add the pink layer ingredients in a blender. Blend for making a smooth liquid.

4. Pour the pink liquid slowly over the orange layer.

5. Pour in such a way so that both layers can be differentiated.

6. Serve immediately.

Ginger, Carrot, and Turmeric Smoothie

Total Prep & Cooking Time: Forty minutes

Yields: Two servings

Nutrition Facts: Calories: 140 | Protein: 2.6g | Carbs: 30.2g | Fat: 2.2g | Fiber: 5.6g

Ingredients

For carrot juice:

- Two cups of water
- Two and a half cups of carrots

For smoothie:

- One ripe banana (sliced)
- One cup of pineapple (frozen, cubed)
- Half tbsp. of ginger
- One-fourth tsp. of turmeric (ground)
- Half cup of carrot juice
- One tbsp. of lemon juice
- One-third cup of almond milk

Method:

1. Add water and carrots in a high power blender. Blend on high settings for making smooth juice.

2. Take a dish towel and strain the juice over a bowl. Squeeze the towel for taking out most of the juice.

3. Add the ingredients for the smoothie in a blender and blend until frothy and creamy.

4. Add carrot juice and blend again.

5. Pour the smoothie in glasses and serve.

Sweet Potato and Mango Smoothie
Total Prep & Cooking Time: Ten minutes

Yields: Two servings

Nutrition Facts: Calories: 133.3 | Protein: 3.6g | Carbs: 28.6g | Fat: 1.3g | Fiber: 6.2g

Ingredients

- One small sweet potato (cooked, smashed)
- Half cup of mango chunks (frozen)
- Two cups of coconut milk
- One tbsp. of chia seeds
- Two tsps. of maple syrup
- A handful of ice cubes

Method:

1. Add mango chunks and sweet potato in a high power blender. Blend until frothy and smooth.

2. Add chia seeds, coconut milk, ice cubes, and maple syrup. Blend again for one minute.

3. Divide the smoothie in glasses and serve.

Carrot Cake Smoothie

Total Prep & Cooking Time: Ten minutes

Yields: Two servings

Nutrition Facts: Calories: 289.3 | Protein: 3.6g | Carbs: 47.8g | Fat: 1.3g | Fiber: 0.6g

Ingredients

- One cup of carrots (chopped)
- One banana
- Half cup of almond milk
- One cup of Greek yogurt
- One tbsp. of maple syrup
- One tsp. of cinnamon (ground)
- One-fourth tsp. of nutmeg
- Half tsp. of ginger (ground)
- A handful of ice cubes

Method

1. Add banana, carrots, and almond milk in a blender. Blend until frothy and smooth.

2. Add yogurt, cinnamon, maple syrup, ginger, nutmeg, and ice cubes. Blend again for two minutes.

3. Divide the smoothie in serving glasses and serve.

Notes:

- You can add more ice cubes and turn the smoothie into slushy.

- You can store the leftover smoothie in the freezer for two days.

Chapter 4: Green Smoothies

Green smoothies can help in the process of detoxification as well as weight loss. Here are some easy-to-make green smoothie recipes for you.

Kale Avocado Smoothie

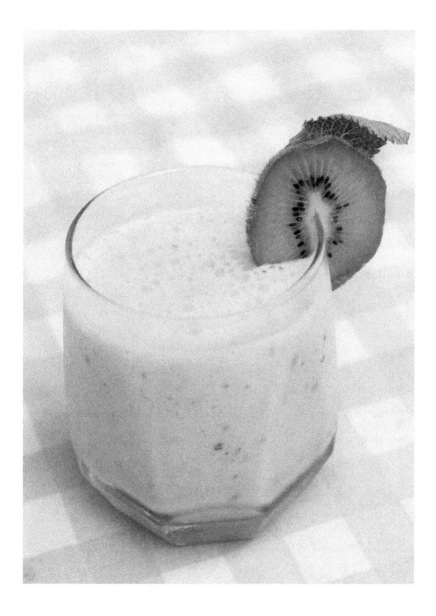

Total Prep & Cooking Time: Ten minutes

Yields: Two servings

Nutrition Facts: Calories: 401 | Protein: 11.2g | Carbs: 64.6g | Fat: 17.3g | Fiber: 10.2g

Ingredients

- One banana (cut in chunks)
- Half cup of blueberry yogurt
- One cup of kale (chopped)
- Half ripe avocado
- One-third cup of almond milk

Method:

1. Add blueberry, banana, avocado, and kale in a blender. Blend for making a smooth mixture.

2. Add the almond milk and blend again.

3. Divide the smoothie in glasses and serve.

Celery Pineapple Smoothie

Total Prep & Cooking Time: Ten minutes

Yields: Two servings

Nutrition Facts: Calories: 112 | Protein: 2.3g | Carbs: 3.6g | Fat: 1.2g | Fiber: 3.9g

Ingredients

- Three celery stalks (chopped)
- One cup of cubed pineapple
- One banana
- One pear
- Half cup of almond milk
- One tsp. of honey

Method:

1. Add celery stalks, pear, banana, and cubes of pineapple in a food processor. Blend until frothy and smooth.

2. Add honey and almond milk. Blend for two minutes.

3. Pour the smoothie in serving glasses and enjoy!

Cucumber Mango and Lime Smoothie

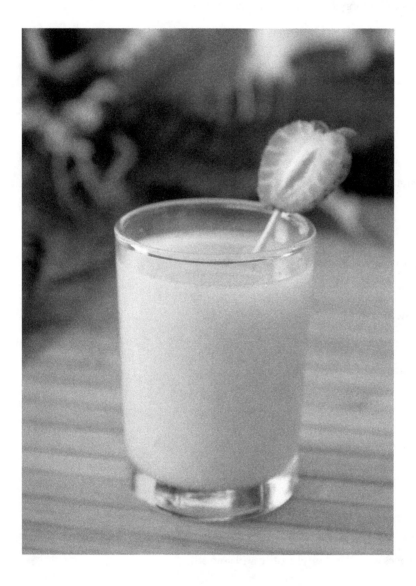

Total Prep & Cooking Time: Ten minutes

Yields: Two servings

Nutrition Facts: Calories: 165 | Protein: 2.2g | Carbs: 32.5g | Fat: 4.2g | Fiber:

3.7g

Ingredients

- One cup of ripe mango (frozen, cubed)
- Six cubes of ice
- Half cup of baby spinach leaves
- Two leaves of mint
- Two tsps. of lime juice
- Half cucumber (chopped)
- Three-fourth cup of coconut milk
- One-eighth tsp. of cayenne pepper

Method:

1. Add mango cubes, spinach leaves, and cucumber in a high power blender. Blend until frothy and smooth.

2. Add mint leaves, lime juice, coconut milk, cayenne pepper, and ice cubes. Process the ingredients until smooth.

3. Pour the smoothie in glasses and serve.

Kale, Melon, and Broccoli Smoothie

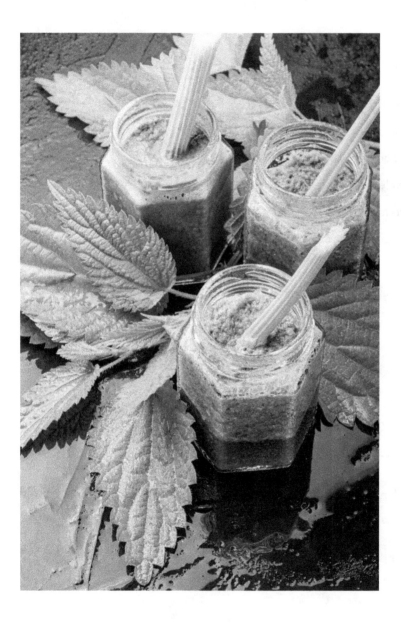

Total Prep & Cooking Time: Ten minutes

Yields: One serving

Nutrition Facts: Calories: 96.3 | Protein: 2.3g | Carbs: 24.3g | Fat: 1.2g | Fiber: 2.6g

Ingredients

- Eight ounces of honeydew melon
- One handful of kale
- Two ounces of broccoli florets
- One cup of coconut water
- Two sprigs of mint
- Two dates
- Half cup of lime juice
- Eight cubes of ice

Method:

1. Add kale, melon, and broccoli in a food processor. Whizz the ingredients for blending.

2. Add mint leaves and coconut water. Blend again.

3. Add lime juice, dates, and ice cubes. Blend the ingredients until smooth and creamy.

4. Pour the smoothie in a smoothie glass. Enjoy!

Kiwi Spinach Smoothie

Total Prep & Cooking Time: Ten minutes

Yields: Two servings

Nutrition Facts: Calories: 102 | Protein: 3.6g | Carbs: 21.3g | Fat: 2.2g | Fiber: 3.1g

Ingredients

- One kiwi (cut in chunks)
- One banana (cut in chunks)
- One cup of spinach leaves
- Three-fourth cup of almond milk
- One tbsp. of chia seeds
- Four cubes of ice

Method:

1. Add banana, kiwi, and spinach leaves in a blender. Blend the ingredients until smooth.

2. Add chia seeds, ice cubes, and almond milk. Blend again for one minute.

3. Pour the smoothie in serving glasses and serve.

Avocado Smoothie

Total Prep & Cooking Time: Ten minutes

Yields: Two servings

Nutrition Facts: Calories: 345 | Protein: 9.1g | Carbs: 47.8g | Fat: 16.9g | Fiber: 6.7g

Ingredients

- One ripe avocado (halved, pitted)
- One cup of milk
- Half cup of vanilla yogurt
- Eight cubes of ice
- Three tbsps. of honey

Method:

1. Add avocado, vanilla yogurt, and milk in a blender. Blend the ingredients until frothy and smooth.

2. Add honey and ice cubes. Blend the ingredients for making a smooth mixture.

3. Serve immediately.

PART IV

Vegetarian Cookbook

The vegetarian diet has gained immense popularity in the last few years. According to some studies, it has been found that an estimated 18% of the world population is vegetarian. Apart from all the environmental and ethical benefits of removing meat from the diet, a properly planned vegetarian diet can reduce the risk of various chronic diseases, improve diet quality, and help in losing weight. The vegetarian diet also does not include poultry and fish. The majority of the people opt for a vegetarian diet for personal or religious reasons and for ethical reasons, such as animal rights. Other people opt for it for various environmental reasons, like livestock production, which results in the emission of greenhouse gases.

A vegetarian diet comes along with a wide array of benefits. It has been found that vegetarians have a better quality of diet when compared to meat-eaters. They also have a higher intake of beneficial nutrients, such as vitamin C, fiber, magnesium, and vitamin E. Switching from a normal meat diet to a vegetarian diet can result to be an effective strategy in case you want to lose weight. For instance, in a review of twelve studies, it has been found that vegetarians can lose about four pounds of weight over eighteen weeks than non-vegetarians. Also, vegetarians have lower BMI or body mass index than non-vegetarians.

Some research found that a vegetarian diet can be linked to a lower risk of developing cancer and those of the colon, breast, stomach, and rectum. However, it lacks enough evidence to prove that a vegetarian diet can effectively reduce cancer risk. People who follow a vegetarian diet can maintain healthy levels of blood sugar. It can also help in preventing the onset of diabetes by controlling the levels of blood sugar. Vegetarian diets help in the reduction of various heart diseases that can make your heart stronger and healthier.

A vegetarian diet needs to include a wide mixture of veggies, fruits, healthy fats, grains, and proteins. To replace the protein that you get from meat in a diet, you will need to include plant foods rich in proteins such as seeds, nuts, legumes, seitan, tofu, and tempeh. Consuming whole foods rich in nutrients, such as vegetables and fruits, can provide your body with the necessary minerals and vitamins to fill the nutritional gaps in a diet. Some of the food items that you can include in your diet are:

- **Fruits:** Bananas, apples, melons, oranges, peaches, pears

- **Vegetables:** Asparagus, leafy greens, carrots, broccoli

- **Legumes:** Beans, lentils, chickpeas, peas

- **Seeds:** Chia, flaxseed, hemp

- **Nuts:** Walnuts, cashews, almonds

- **Proteins:** Seitan, natto, tofu, eggs, tempeh

You cannot include food items such as fish, seafood, meat, poultry, and ingredients that are based on meat. Restriction of eggs and dairy products are applicable for the vegans and not for vegetarians. I have included some tasty and easy vegetarian recipes that will help you to plan your diet effectively.

Chapter 1: Breakfast Recipes

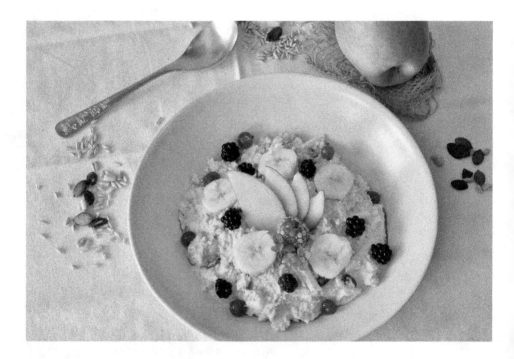

No matter which diet you follow, breakfast is very important in all cases. In this section, you will find some easy-to-make and tasty breakfast recipes that you can include in your vegetarian diet.

Black Bean Bowl

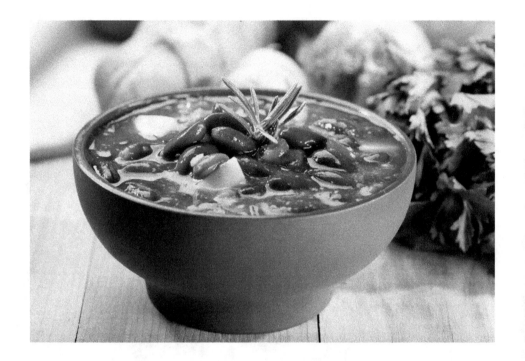

Total Prep & Cooking Time: Fifteen minutes

Yields: Two servings

Nutrition Facts: Calories: 620.1 | Protein: 28.9g | Carbs: 47.6g | Fat: 37.1g | Fiber: 23.2g

Ingredients:

- Two tbsps. of olive oil

- Four eggs (beaten)
- One can of black beans (rinsed)
- One avocado (sliced)
- One-fourth cup of salsa
- One tsp. of each
  - Black pepper (ground)
  - Salt

Method:

1. Take a small pan and heat oil in it. Add the eggs and scramble for five minutes.

2. Place the beans in a bowl. Heat the beans in the oven for one minute.

3. Divide the beans into two serving bowls.

4. Top the beans with scrambled eggs, salsa, and avocado. Add pepper and salt according to taste.

Coconut Blueberry Ricotta Bowl

Total Prep & Cooking Time: Twenty minutes

Yields: One serving

Nutrition Facts: Calories: 303.2 | Protein: 9.5g | Carbs: 32.1g | Fat: 15.3g | Fiber: 3.9g

Ingredients:

- One-fourth cup of ricotta cheese
- One tbsp. of each
  - Honey
  - Coconut milk
  - Slivered almonds
  - Coconut flakes
- Half cup of blueberries

Method:

1. Combine coconut milk and ricotta in a medium-sized bowl. Drizzle honey from the top and add coconut and almonds.

2. Serve with blueberries from the top.

Broccoli Quiche

Total Prep & Cooking Time: Fifty minutes

Yields: Six servings

Nutrition Facts: Calories: 378.2 | Protein: 17.3g | Carbs: 21.1g | Fat: 25.8g | Fiber: 3.1g

Ingredients:

- One pie crust (unbaked)
- Three tbsps. of butter
- One onion (minced)
- One tsp. of each
  - Garlic (minced)
  - Salt
- Two cups of broccoli (chopped)
- One and a half cup of mozzarella cheese (shredded)
- Four eggs (beaten)
- Two and a half cup of milk
- Half tsp. of black pepper
- One tbsp. of butter (melted)

Method

;

1. Start by preheating your oven at 175 degrees Celsius. Use pie crust for lining a deep pie pan.

2. Take a large saucepan and add butter to it. Add broccoli, onion, and garlic. Cook the veggies slowly until tender. Add the cooked veggies to the pie crust and add cheese from the top.

3. Mix milk and eggs in a bowl; add pepper and salt for seasoning. Add the remaining butter to the milk mixture. Pour the mixture over the mixture of vegetables.

4. Bake the quiche in the oven for forty minutes or until the center has properly set.

Tomato Bagel Sandwich

Total Prep & Cooking Time: Twenty minutes

Yields: One serving

Nutrition Facts: Calories: 346.3 | Protein: 13.1g | Carbs: 48.6g | Fat: 10.7g | Fiber: 2.9g

Ingredients:

- One bagel (split, toasted)
- Two tbsps. of cream cheese
- One large tomato (sliced thinly)
- Pepper and salt (to season)
- Four basil leaves

Method:

1. Spread the cream cheese on the halves of the bagel.

2. Top the cheese layer with slices of tomato. Add pepper and salt for seasoning.

3. Serve with basil leaves from the top.

Cornmeal And Blueberry Pancakes

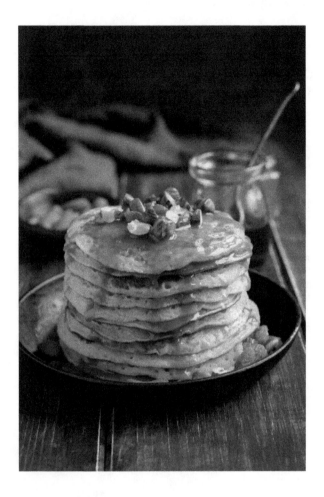

Total Prep & Cooking Time: Thirty minutes

Yields: Six servings

Nutrition Facts: Calories: 180.3 | Protein: 5.2g | Carbs: 26.8g | Fat: 5.1g | Fiber: 4.6g

Ingredients:

- One cup of soy milk
- Half cup of each
    - Water
    - Cornmeal (ground)
- One and a half cup of wheat flour
- One tsp. baking powder
- One-third tsp. baking soda
- One-fourth tsp. of salt
- One cup of blueberries
- Two tbsps. of vegetable oil

Method:

1. Preheat your oven at 95 degrees Celsius.

2. Combine water and soy milk in a bowl.

3. Take a large mixing bowl and combine cornmeal, baking soda, flour, salt, and baking powder. Add the mixture of soy milk. Combine properly. Add the blueberries and allow the batter to rest for five minutes.

4. Take a large skillet and grease it using oil. Add one-fourth cup of the batter in the skillet. Cook until the pancakes are bubbly on the top, and the edges are dry. Cook for five minutes on each side. Repeat with the remaining batter.

5. Serve hot with jam or syrup.

Breakfast Tortilla

Total Prep & Cooking Time: Twenty minutes

Yields: Two servings

Nutrition Facts: Calories: 381.3 | Protein: 15.8g | Carbs: 38.1g | Fat: 18.7g | Fiber: 4.5g

Ingredients:

- Two tbsps. of beans (refried)
- Three tbsps. of salsa
- Three large eggs (beaten)
- One tbsp. of mayonnaise
- Four tortillas (flour)
- One and a half cup of lettuce (shredded)

Method:

1. Combine salsa and beans in a small bowl.

2. Take an iron skillet and heat oil in it. Add the eggs and let the bottom set—Cook for one minute. Spread the mixture of beans on half of the egg and flip one side for making the shape of a half-circle. Cook until the eggs set properly.

3. Spread mayonnaise on the tortillas.

4. Cut the cooked eggs into four equal pieces. Place each piece of eggs on the tortillas. Top with lettuce.

5. Roll the tortillas. Serve hot.

Zucchini Frittata

Total Prep & Cooking Time: Forty minutes

Yields: Five servings

Nutrition Facts: Calories: 258.3 | Protein: 14.2g | Carbs: 9.1g | Fat: 19.6g | Fiber: 3.4g

Ingredients:

- One cup of water
- Three tbsps. of olive oil
- Half tsp. of salt
- Half bell pepper (green, chopped)
- Three zucchinis (cut in slices of half-inch)
- Two garlic cloves (peeled)
- One onion (diced)
- Six mushrooms (chopped)
- One tbsp. of butter
- Five eggs
- Pepper and salt (to taste)
- One and a half cup of mozzarella cheese (shredded)
- Three tbsps. of parmesan cheese

Method:

1. Start by preheating your oven at 160/175 degrees Celsius.

2. Take a large skillet and combine olive oil, water, green pepper, salt, garlic cloves, and zucchini. Simmer the mixture until the zucchini is soft—Cook for seven minutes.

3. Drain the water and remove the garlic; add mushroom, onion, and butter. Keep cooking until the onion turns transparent. Add the eggs and keep stirring. Add pepper and salt for seasoning. Cook until the eggs are firm.

4. Add mozzarella cheese from the top.

5. Bake in the oven for ten minutes.

6. Remove the frittata from the oven and add parmesan cheese from the top. Place under the broiler for about five minutes.

7. Cut the frittata in wedges and serve warm.

Oatmeal And Strawberry Smoothie

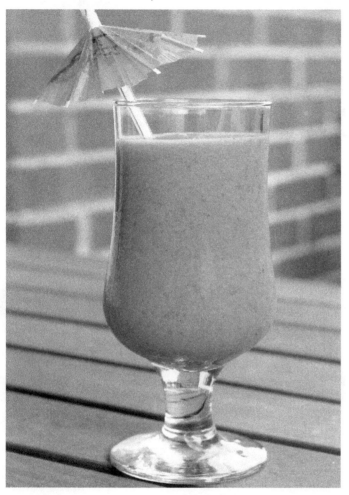

Total Prep & Cooking Time: Twenty minutes

Yields: Two servings

Nutrition Facts: Calories: 204.1 | Protein: 5.2g | Carbs: 41.3g | Fat: 2.7g | Fiber: 6.9g

Ingredients:

- One cup of almond milk
- Half cup of rolled oats
- Fourteen strawberries (frozen)
- One banana (cut in chunks)
- Two tsps. of agave nectar
- Half tsp. of vanilla extract

Method:

1. Add almond milk, strawberries, oats, agave nectar, banana, and vanilla extract in a food processor. Keep blending until smooth.

2. Serve with pieces of strawberry from the top.

Chapter 2: Appetizers Recipes

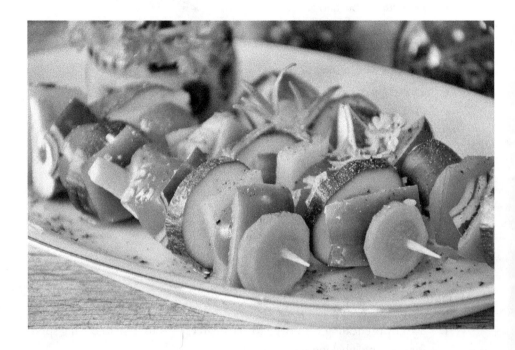

Hosting a party but not sure which appetizers to prepare as most of your guests are vegetarians? No worries as I have included some great vegetarian recipes for appetizers in this section.

Buffalo Cauliflower
Total Prep & Cooking Time: Thirty minutes

Yields: Twelve servings

Nutrition Facts: Calories: 120 | Protein: 4.2g | Carbs: 7.9g | Fat: 8.7g | Fiber: 2.3g

Ingredients:

- One serving of cooking spray
- Half cup of buffalo sauce
- Three tbsps. of mayonnaise
- One large egg
- Six cups of cauliflower florets
- Two cups of garlic croutons
- One-fourth cup of parmesan cheese (grated)

For the dipping sauce:

- One-fourth cup of each
  - Sour cream
  - Blue cheese salad dressing
- One tsp. of black pepper (ground)
-

Method:

1. Start by preheating your oven to 230 degrees Celsius. Use a cooking spray for greasing a baking tray.

2. Combine mayonnaise, buffalo sauce, and egg in a bowl. Toss the florets of cauliflower in the mixture of sauce and coat properly.

3. Spread the tossed florets on the baking tray.

4. Add the croutons on a blender and pulse them into crumbs. Add the cheese and pulse again. Spread the mixture of cheese and croutons over the florets of cauliflower.

5. Bake for fifteen minutes until tender and browned. Allow the florets to sit for five minutes.

6. Mix all the ingredients for the dipping sauce.

7. Serve cauliflower florets with dip sauce by the side.

Garlic Bread And Veggie Delight

Total Prep & Cooking Time: Thirty minutes

Yields: Five servings

Nutrition Facts: Calories: 390.2 | Protein: 12.4g | Carbs: 58.7g | Fat: 11.6g | Fiber: 7.2g

Ingredients:

- One cup of olive oil
- One garlic clove (chopped)
- One eggplant (cubed)
- One zucchini (cubed)
- One tomato (chopped)
- One tsp. of salt
- Two tsps. of each
    - Basil (minced)
    - Oregano (minced)
- One baguette
- Four tsps. of garlic powder
- Six tsps. of butter

Method:

1. Take a large skillet and add olive oil to it. Add garlic and fry for two minutes until browned.

2. Add the zucchini and eggplant to the skillet and cook for five minutes. Make sure that the eggplant is tender and brown.

3. Add the chunks of tomato and combine the veggies; add basil, oregano, and salt. Cook for two minutes and remove from heat.

4. Preheat oven 140/165 degrees Celsius.

5. Slice the baguette into one-inch slices, approximately twelve slices. Add butter and garlic powder on the bread slices and place them on the oven rack. Heat the bread for five minutes.

6. Arrange the heated bread slices on a plate. Top the slices with vegetables.

7. Serve immediately.

Spinach Parmesan Balls

Total Prep & Cooking Time: Thirty minutes

Yields: Ten servings

Nutrition Facts: Calories: 254.1 | Protein: 11.4g | Carbs: 18.4g | Fat: 14.2g | Fiber: 3.5g

Ingredients:

- Twenty ounces of frozen spinach (chopped)
- Two cups of bread crumbs
- One cup of parmesan cheese (grated)
- Half cup of butter (melted)
- Four green onions (chopped)
- Four eggs (beaten)
- Pepper and salt (for seasoning)

Method:

1. Start by preheating your oven at 175 degrees Celsius.

2. Take a bowl and combine spinach, bread crumbs, cheese, green onions, butter, pepper, salt, and eggs. Make balls of one-inch size from the prepared mixture.

3. Arrange the spinach balls on a baking tray. Bake for fifteen minutes until browned.

4. Serve hot.

Cheese Garlic Bread

Total Prep & Cooking Time: Thirty minutes

Yields: Eight servings

Nutrition Facts: Calories: 260 | Protein: 7.1g | Carbs: 29.7g | Fat: 11.4g | Fiber: 1.5g

Ingredients:

- Half cup of butter (melted)
- One tsp. of garlic salt
- One-fourth tsp. of rosemary (dried)
- One-eighth tsp. of each
  - Basil (dried)
  - Thyme (dried)
  - Garlic powder
- One tbsp. of parmesan cheese (grated)
- One loaf of French bread (halved)

Method:

1. Preheat oven at 150 degrees Celsius.

2. Mix garlic salt, butter, basil, rosemary, thyme, garlic powder, and cheese in a bowl.

3. Spread the butter mixture on the halves of the bread. Add extra cheese from the top if you want to.

4. Place halves of bread on a baking tray. Bake for twelve minutes until browned.

Stuffed Mushrooms

Total Prep & Cooking Time: Forty-five minutes

Yields: Twelve servings

Nutrition Facts: Calories: 89 | Protein: 2.6g | Carbs: 1.3g | Fat: 8.9g | Fiber: 0.6g

Ingredients:

- Twelve whole mushrooms
- One tbsp. of each
  - Minced garlic
  - Vegetable oil
- Eight ounces of cream cheese (softened)
- One-fourth cup of parmesan cheese (grated)
- One-fourth tsp. of each
  - Onion powder
  - Black pepper (ground)
  - Cayenne powder (ground)

Method:

1. Preheat the oven to 175 degrees Celsius. Grease a baking tray with the help of cooking spray.

2. Clean the mushrooms using a damp kitchen towel; break the stems. Chop the mushroom stems finely.

3. Take a skillet and heat oil in it. Add chopped stems of mushroom and garlic—Cook for five minutes.

4. Remove the skillet from heat and let it cool. Add the cream cheese, black pepper, parmesan cheese, cayenne powder, and onion powder. Mix well.

5. Use a small spoon for filling the mushroom caps with the mushroom stuffing.

6. Place the mushroom caps on the prepared baking tray.

7. Bake for twenty minutes until liquid forms under the mushroom caps.

Tomato Bruschetta

Total Prep & Cooking Time: Thirty-five minutes

Yields: Twelve servings

Nutrition Facts: Calories: 214.1 | Protein: 10.6g | Carbs: 23.1g | Fat: 8.8g | Fiber: 2.6g

Ingredients:

- Six tomatoes (chopped)
- Half cup of sun-dried tomatoes
- Three garlic cloves (minced)
- One-fourth cup of olive oil
- Two tbsps. of balsamic vinegar
- One-third cup of basil
- One-fourth tsp. of each
    o Black pepper (ground)
    o Salt
- One baguette
- Two cups of mozzarella cheese (shredded)

Method:

1. Preheat your oven on the setting of broiler.

2. Combine tomatoes, olive oil, vinegar, garlic, sun-dried tomatoes, basil, pepper, and salt in a bowl. Let the mixture sit for ten minutes.

3. Cut the baguette into slices of a three-fourth inch. Arrange the baguette slices on a baking tray. Broil for two minutes until browned.

4. Add the mixture of tomatoes on the slices of bread and top with mozzarella cheese.

5. Broil again for five minutes.

Spicy Pumpkin Seeds

Total Prep & Cooking Time: One hour and ten minutes

Yields: Eight servings

Nutrition Facts: Calories: 91 | Protein: 3.2g | Carbs: 8.8g | Fat: 4.9g | Fiber: 0.7g

Ingredients:

- Two tbsps. of margarine
- Half tsp. of salt
- One-eighth tsp. of garlic salt
- Two tsps. of Worcestershire sauce
- Two cups of pumpkin seeds (raw)

Method:

1. Preheat your oven at 135 degrees Celsius.

2. Combine the ingredients in a mixing bowl.

3. Bake for one hour. Stir in between.

Chapter 3: Soups & Side Dishes Recipes

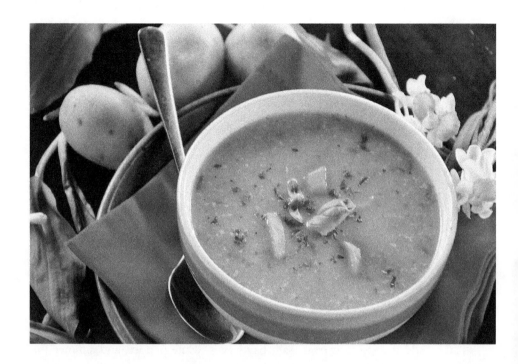

Soup forms an integral part of a vegetarian diet along with the side dishes. Here are some easy vegetarian recipes for side dishes and soups that you can include in your diet.

Carrot Soup
Total Prep & Cooking Time: Forty-five minutes

Yields: Four servings

Nutrition Facts: Calories: 351 | Protein: 3.2g | Carbs: 23.1g | Fat: 29.7g | Fiber: 4.2g

Ingredients:

- Two tbsps. of olive oil
- Four-hundred grams of carrots (cut in disks of half-inch)
- Half onion (diced)
- Four cloves of garlic (smashed)
- Two tsps. of cumin seeds
- Four cups of vegetable stock
- Two bay leaves
- One tsp. of salt
- One-fourth tsp. of white pepper
- Two tsps. of honey
- One-fourth cup of yogurt

Method:

1. Take a heavy bottom pan and add oil in it. Add onions, garlic, and cumin to the pan. Sauté on a medium flame for six minutes until tender and golden in color. Stir occasionally.

2. Add the stock, carrots, salt, bay leaves, white pepper, and simmer the mixture. Cover the pan and simmer for twenty minutes. Allow the soup to cool down for five minutes.

3. Use an immersion blender for blending the soup. Blend until you reach a silky smooth consistency.

4. Return the soup to heat and add honey. Stir the soup. Add yogurt and simmer. Taste the soup and adjust the seasonings. Keep the soup warm on very low flame until you serve.

5. Divide the soup among serving bowls. Serve with a dollop of yogurt from the top.

Note: You can use ground spices in place of the whole spices. But, whole spices will help in adding extra flavor.

Celery Soup

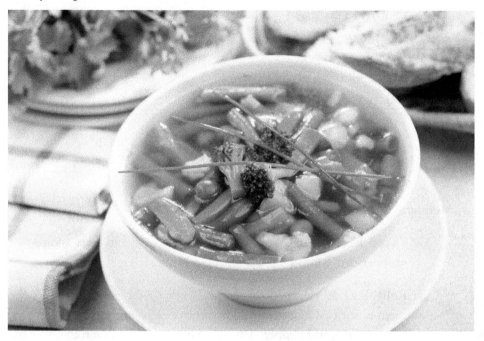

Total Prep & Cooking Time: Thirty-five minutes

Yields: Seven servings

Nutrition Facts: Calories: 180 | Protein: 4.2g | Carbs: 23.1g | Fat: 9.2g | Fiber: 4.9g

Ingredients:

- Two tbsps. of olive oil
- One onion (diced)
- Four cloves of garlic (chopped)
- Six cups of celery (thinly sliced)
- Two cups of potatoes (sliced in rounds)
- Four cups of vegetable stock

- One cup of water
- One bay leaf
- One tsp. of salt
- Half tsp. of pepper
- One-third tsp. of cayenne
- Half cup of sour cream
- One-fourth cup of each
  - Parsley (small stems)
  - Dill (small stems)

Method:

1. Take a large pot and add oil in it. Heat the oil and start adding the onion. Cook for five minutes until golden.

2. Roughly chop celery, potatoes, and garlic. Add garlic and cook the mixture for two minutes. Add potatoes, celery, stock, bay leaf, water, salt, cayenne, and pepper. The liquid needs to be enough to cover the vegetables. Cover the pot and boil the mixture. Simmer for ten minutes.

3. Remove bay leaf after turning off the stove. Add herbs to the pot and allow them to wilt.

4. Take an immersion blender and start blending the soup until silky smooth.

5. Return the pot to heat and cook over low flame for five minutes.

6. Serve with sour cream from the top.

Tomato Soup And Halloumi Croutons

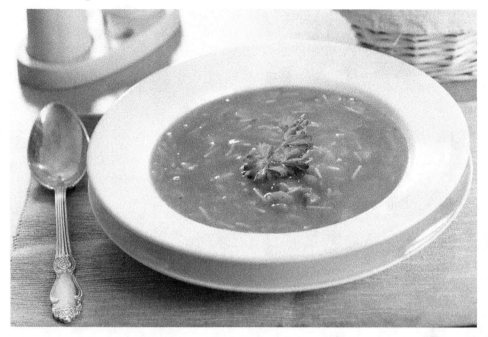

Total Prep & Cooking Time: One hour and five minutes

Yields: Six servings

Nutrition Facts: Calories: 285 | Protein: 10.3g | Carbs: 13.2g | Fat: 23.2g | Fiber: 4.9g

Ingredients:

- Three pounds of tomatoes
- Half red onion (sliced in thin rings)
- Six cloves of garlic
- Two tsps. of thyme leaves

- One-third cup of oil
- Four cups of vegetable stock
- One-fourth cup of basil leaves (chopped)
- One cup of Greek yogurt

For croutons:

- One block of halloumi cheese (cut in cubes of three-fourth inch)
- One tbsp. of oil

Method:

1. Start by preheating your oven at 200 degrees Celsius.

2. Use parchment paper for lining baking sheet. Spread the onions, tomatoes, and garlic on the sheet. Drizzle with some oil from the top—roast in the oven for thirty minutes.

3. Heat some oil in a pan and start adding the halloumi cubes. Cook for four minutes until golden on all sides.

4. Add the roasted veggies in a pot along with the vegetable stock. Use an immersion blender for blending the soup until smooth. Place the pot over a low flame and add seasonings of your choice. Simmer the soup and add basil. Simmer for ten minutes.

5. Add half a cup of yogurt to the soup.

6. Serve the soup in serving bowls with croutons from the top.

Baked Potatoes And Mushrooms With Spinach

Total Prep & Cooking Time: Forty-five minutes

Yields: Four servings

Nutrition Facts: Calories: 235.1 | Protein: 7.1g | Carbs: 27.1g | Fat: 11.3g | Fiber: 4.9g

Ingredients:

- One pound of potatoes (halved)
- Three tbsps. of olive oil
- Half pound of Portobello mushroom
- Six garlic cloves
- Two tbsps. of thyme (chopped)
- One pinch of black pepper and salt
- One-fourth cup of cherry tomatoes
- Half cup of spinach (sliced)
- Two tbsps. of pine nuts (toasted)

Method:

1. Preheat your oven at 200/220 degrees Celsius.

2. Add the potatoes in a roasting pan and drizzle some oil from the top. Roast the potatoes for fifteen minutes.

3. Add mushrooms along with garlic to the pan. Add thyme from the top along with some olive oil. Sprinkle black pepper and salt. Roast again for five minutes.

4. Add cherry tomatoes to the pan. Cook again for five minutes until the mushrooms are tender.

5. Add toasted pine nuts from the top and serve with spinach by the side.

Garlic Potatoes

Total Prep & Cooking Time: Fifty minutes

Yields: Four servings

Nutrition Facts: Calories: 270.2 | Protein: 5.2g | Carbs: 39.7g | Fat: 12.1g | Fiber: 4.9g

Ingredients:

- Two pounds of red potatoes (quartered)
- One-fourth cup of butter (melted)
- Two tsps. of garlic (minced)
- One tsp. of salt
- One lemon (juiced)
- One tbsp. of parmesan cheese (grated)

Method:

1. Start by preheating the oven at 175 degrees Celsius.

2. Place the potatoes in a baking dish.

3. Combine butter, lemon juice, garlic, and salt in a small bowl. Add this mixture over the potatoes and stir for coating. Add parmesan cheese from the top.

4. Bake the potatoes by covering the dish in the preheated oven for thirty minutes. Remove the cover and bake again for ten minutes.

Buttery Carrots

Total Prep & Cooking Time: Twenty-five minutes

Yields: Four servings

Nutrition Facts: Calories: 182.3 | Protein: 0.8g | Carbs: 21.3g | Fat: 10.3g | Fiber: 3.9g

Ingredients:

- One pound of baby carrots
- One-fourth cup of margarine
- One-third cup of brown sugar

Method:

1. Cook the baby carrots in boiling water. Drain most of the liquid leaving behind a little bit of liquid at the base.

2. Remove the carrots from the pot. Add brown sugar along with margarine. Simmer the mixture for two minutes and add the carrots to the pot. Toss well for combining.

3. Serve warm.

Chapter 4: Main Course Recipes

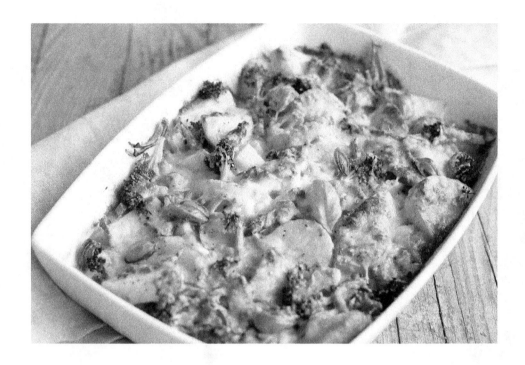

After you are done with the soups and side dishes, now it is time to jump into the main course. Here are some tasty main course recipes that you can include within your vegetarian diet plan.

Nut And Tofu Loaf

Total Prep & Cooking Time: One hour and forty minutes

Yields: Six servings

Nutrition Facts: Calories: 308.3 | Protein: 15.2g | Carbs: 27.6g | Fat: 14.2g | Fiber: 4.8g

Ingredients:

- One serving of cooking spray
- Twelve ounces of tofu (firm, drained, cubed)
- Two large eggs
- One ounce dry mix of onion soup
- One tbsp. of soy sauce
- Three-fourth cup of walnuts (chopped)
- One tsp. of olive oil
- Eight ounces of fresh mushrooms (sliced)
- One onion (chopped)
- Two celery stalks (chopped)
- Two tsps. of oregano (dried)
- One and a half tsps. of basil (dried)
- Half tsp. of sage (dried)
- Two cups of bread crumbs

Method:

1. Start by preheating the oven at 175 degrees Celsius. Use a cooking spray for greasing loaf pan.

2. Place eggs, tofu, soy sauce, and onion soup mix in a blender. Blend the ingredients until properly combined. Add the walnuts and blend again. Transfer the mixture of tofu to a bowl.

3. Take a large skillet and heat oil in it. Add mushrooms and cook them for four minutes. Add celery and cook for two minutes—season with basil, sage, and oregano.

4. Stir bread crumbs and veggies into the mixture of tofu. Press the loaf mixture into the pan.

5. Bake the loaf in the oven for sixty to seventy minutes.

6. Let the loaf cool down for five minutes before serving.

7. Slice the loaf and serve warm.

Velvety Chickpea Curry

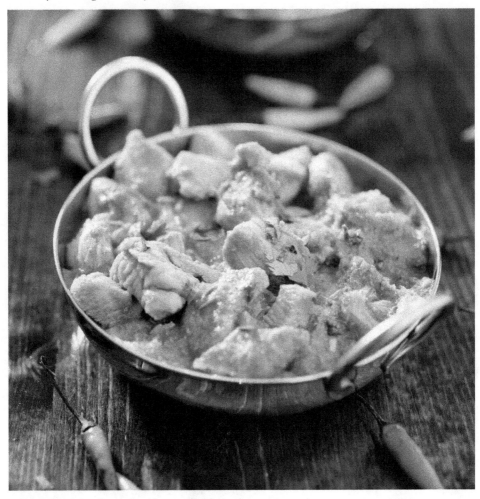

Total Prep & Cooking Time: Forty-five minutes

Yields: Six servings

Nutrition Facts: Calories: 408.3 | Protein: 10.2g | Carbs: 68.3g | Fat: 11.2g | Fiber: 8.9g

Ingredients:

- One tbsp. of each
    - Ginger root (minced)
    - Coconut oil
- One onion (sliced)
- Four garlic cloves (minced)
- Two tbsps. of curry powder
- One-fourth tsp. of pepper flakes
- Three cups of vegetable stock
- Two tbsps. of each
    - Soy sauce
    - Tomato paste
    - Maple syrup
- Half pound of potatoes (cut in pieces of a three-fourth inch)
- One carrot (sliced)
- Four cups of cauliflower florets
- One can of chickpeas (rinsed)
- Half cup of coconut milk
- One-fourth cup of cilantro (chopped)
- Half cup of peas (frozen)
- Salt (for seasoning)

Method:

1. Take a heavy-based pot and melt coconut oil in it. Add onions to the pot and sauté for five minutes. Add garlic and ginger to the pot—Cook for thirty seconds. Add pepper flakes, curry powder, soy sauce, stock, tomato paste, and maple syrup. Stir well.

2. Add carrots and potatoes to the pot and cover. Boil the mixture. Slightly open the cover and simmer for ten minutes. Add chickpeas, cauliflower, cilantro, and coconut milk. Stir well for combining. Simmer again for seven minutes. Add peas and cook for one minute.

3. Season with salt and cook for one minute.

4. Serve with basmati rice and cilantro from the top.

Tofu Pad Thai

Total Prep & Cooking Time: Forty-five minutes

Yields: Four servings

Nutrition Facts: Calories: 451 | Protein: 15.4g | Carbs: 60.1g | Fat: 15.2g | Fiber: 4.2g

Ingredients:

- Twelve ounces of tofu (drained, cubed)
- One tbsp. of cornstarch
- Three tbsps. of vegetable oil
- Eight ounces of rice noodles

For the sauce:

- One-fourth cup of each
  - Sriracha sauce
  - Water
  - Soy sauce
- Two tbsps. of white sugar
- One tbsp. of tamarind concentrate
- One tsp. of pepper flakes
- One large egg

- Two tbsps. of spring onions (chopped)
- One and a half tbsp. of peanuts (crushed)
- One lime (cut in wedges)

Method:

1. Coat the tofu cubes with cornstarch in a large bowl.

2. Heat two tbsps. of oil in a skillet. Fry the coated tofu for two minutes on each side.

3. Place the rice noodles in a medium bowl. Cover the noodles using hot boiling water. Soak the noodles until soft for three minutes. Drain the water.

4. Mix sriracha sauce, water, sugar, soy sauce, pepper flakes, and tamarind concentrate in a skillet. Cook for five minutes.

5. Heat one tbsp. of oil in a large wok. Add noodles, onion, along with the tofu. Cook the mixture for three minutes. Add sauce and toss it for combining.

6. Push the noodles to a side and crack the egg in the center. Stir for thirty seconds and mix with the noodles.

7. Serve with peanuts, green onion, and wedges of lime.

Eggplant Parmesan

Total Prep & Cooking Time: One hour

Yields: Ten servings

Nutrition Facts: Calories: 480.2 | Protein: 21.2g | Carbs: 60.1g | Fat: 15.2g | Fiber: 9.8g

Ingredients:

- Three eggplants (sliced)
- Two eggs (beaten)
- Four cups of bread crumbs
- Six cups of spaghetti sauce
- Sixteen ounces of mozzarella cheese (shredded)
- Half cup of parmesan cheese
- Half tsp. of basil (dried)

Method:

1. Preheat the oven at 175 degrees Celsius.

2. Dip the slices of eggplant in egg and then coat in bread crumbs.

3. Arrange the slices of eggplant in a baking sheet and bake for five minutes on both sides.

4. Take a baking dish and spread the spaghetti sauce for covering the base. Arrange the eggplant slices over the sauce. Sprinkle cheese from the top. Repeat for the remaining layers. Top with basil and cheese.

5. Bake for thirty-minutes until browned.

Veg Korma
Total Prep & Cooking Time: Fifty-five minutes

Yields: Four servings

Nutrition Facts: Calories: 451 | Protein: 8.4g | Carbs: 40.1g | Fat: 30.2g | Fiber: 8.7g

Ingredients:

- Two tbsps. of vegetable oil
- One onion (diced)
- One tsp. of ginger root (minced)
- Four garlic cloves (minced)
- Two potatoes (cubed)
- Four carrots (cubed)
- One jalapeno pepper (sliced)
- Three tbsps. of cashews (ground)
- One can of tomato sauce
- Two tsps. of salt
- One and a half tbsps. of curry powder
- One cup of green peas (frozen)
- One red bell pepper (roughly chopped)
- One-third yellow bell pepper (roughly chopped)
- One bunch of cilantro
- Half cup of heavy cream

Method:

1. Take a skillet and heat oil in it. Add onions to the oil and cook until soft. Add garlic and ginger to the skillet. Cook for one minute. Add carrots, potatoes, cashews, jalapenos, and tomato sauce. Add curry powder and season with salt. Stir well and cook for ten minutes until the potatoes are soft.

2. Add bell pepper, peas, and cream. Lower the flame and cover the skillet—Cook for ten minutes.

3. Serve with cilantro from the top.

Mac And Cheese
Total Prep & Cooking Time: Fifty minutes

Yields: Six servings

Nutrition Facts: Calories: 456 | Protein: 24g | Carbs: 33.1g | Fat: 24.9g | Fiber: 2.3g

Ingredients:

- Two cups of elbow macaroni (uncooked)
- One-fourth cup of butter
- Two tbsps. of flour
- One tsp. of each
  - Black pepper (ground)
  - Mustard powder
- Two cups of milk
- Eight ounces of each
  - Cheese food (cubed)
  - American cheese (cubed)
- Half cup of bread crumbs

Method:

1. Preheat the oven at 180/200 degrees Celsius. Take a casserole dish and grease with butter.

2. Boil water in a pot with salt. Add the pasta and cook the pasta for six minutes. Drain the water.

3. Take a saucepan. Melt butter in it. Add mustard powder, flour, and pepper. Add milk and stir constantly. Add the cheeses and mix for two minutes until the sauce thickens.

4. Add the macaroni to the cheese mixture. Mix well.

5. Transfer the pasta mixture to the greased dish. Add bread crumbs from the top.

6. Bake for twenty minutes by covering the dish.

7. Serve hot.

Sesame Noodles

Total Prep & Cooking Time: Thirty minutes

Yields: Eight servings

Nutrition Facts: Calories: 365.2 | Protein: 7.3g | Carbs: 51.1g | Fat: 13.2g | Fiber: 3.9g

Ingredients:

- Sixteen ounces of linguine pasta
- Six garlic cloves (minced)
- Six tbsps. of each
    - Safflower oil
    - Sugar
    - Rice vinegar
    - Soy sauce
- Two tsps. of chili sauce
- Two tbsps. of sesame oil
- Six green onions (sliced)
- One tsp. of sesame seeds (toasted)

Method:

1. Boil water in a large pot along with some salt. Add the pasta. Keep cooking for eight minutes. Drain all the water.

2. Take a saucepan and heat oil in it. Add garlic, sugar, soy sauce, chili sauce, and sesame oil. Boil the mixture until the sugar gets dissolved.

3. Add the sauce to the cooked pasta and toss well for combining.

4. Serve with sesame seeds and green onions from the top.

Chapter 5: Dessert Recipes

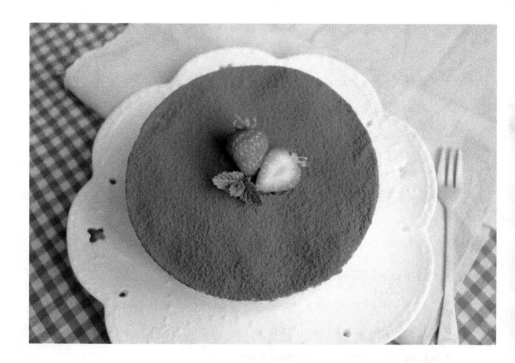

Having a great dessert after a tasty meal can make you, as well as your stomach, feel good. So, here are some vegetarian dessert recipes for you.

Raspberry And Rosewater Sponge Cake

Total Prep & Cooking Time: Fifty-five minutes

Yields: Ten servings

Nutrition Facts: Calories: 441 | Protein: 4.1g | Carbs: 51.3g | Fat: 23.1g | Fiber: 1.3g

Ingredients:

- Two-hundred grams of butter (softened)
- Two-hundred and fifty grams of caster sugar
- Four eggs (beaten)
- One tsp. of vanilla extract
- Two cups of flour

For the rose filling:

- Half cup of double cream
- One tsp. of rosewater
- Four tbsps. of raspberry jam
- One-third cup of raspberries (crushed)

For rose icing:

- Half cup of icing sugar
- Half tsp. of rosewater

Method:

1. Heat the oven at 160 degrees Celsius.

2. Use parchment paper for lining two baking tins—grease with butter.

3. Mix sugar and butter in a bowl. Add the eggs and mix again.

4. Add vanilla extract to the egg mixture and mix. Add flour and fold.

5. Divide the cake batter into the prepared baking tins and bake in the oven for twenty minutes. Let the cakes cool for ten minutes.

6. Whisk double cream along with rosewater. Add the jam and mix.

7. Place one of the cakes on a serving plate and add the cream mixture. Add raspberries from the top and place the other cake on top.

8. Mix all the ingredients for the icing.

9. Serve the cake with rose icing from the top.

Easy Tiramisu

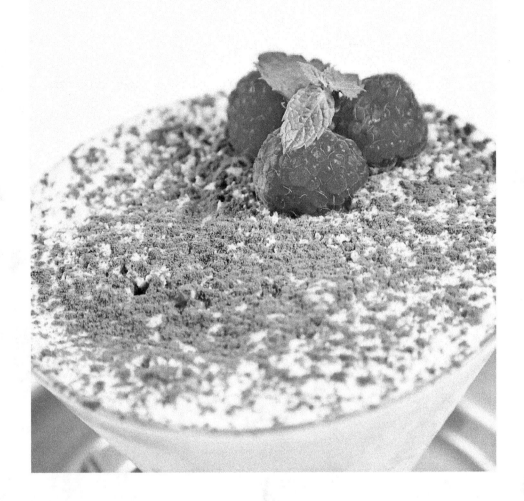

Total Prep & Cooking Time: One hour and fifteen minutes

Yields: Two servings

Nutrition Facts: Calories: 741 | Protein: 11.3g | Carbs: 44.3g | Fat: 51.6g | Fiber: 1.9g

Ingredients:

- Three tsps. of coffee granules
- Three tbsps. of coffee liqueur
- One and a half cup of mascarpone
- Half cup of condensed milk
- Six sponge fingers
- One tbsp. of cocoa powder

Method:

1. Mix coffee granules in two tbsps. of boiling water and stir for combining. Add three tbsps. of cold water along with coffee liqueur. Pour the mixture in a dish and keep aside.

2. Beat condensed milk, mascarpone, and vanilla extract in a bowl using a hand blender.

3. Break the fingers into two pieces and soak them in the mixture of coffee for thirty seconds.

4. Take a sundae glass and add the sponge fingers at the base. Add the cream mixture on top. Sift cocoa powder and chill in the refrigerator for one hour.

Chocolate Marquise

Total Prep & Cooking Time: Two hours and fifty-five minutes

Yields: Ten servings

Nutrition Facts: Calories: 710.3 | Protein: 7.8g | Carbs: 59.8g | Fat: 53g | Fiber: 1.5g

Ingredients:

- Three-hundred grams of dark chocolate
- Half cup of each
  - Caster sugar
  - Butter (softened)
- Six tbsps. of cocoa powder
- Six eggs
- One-third cup of double cream
- One-fourth cup of mint chocolate

Method:

1. Break the dark chocolate in small pieces and melt it using a double boiler system.

2. Beat butter and sugar in a bowl until creamy.

3. Separate the egg whites and yolks.

4. Mix the yolks with the sugar mixture until creamy.

5. Whip the double cream in another bowl.

6. Add the melted chocolate in the mixture of butter and fold gently. Add the whipped cream and mix well.

7. Spoon the mixture of chocolate in a piping bag.

8. Take a baking tin and pipe one layer of chocolate at the base of the tin. Cover the tin with pieces of mint chocolate. Repeat for the other layers. You will need to make four layers of mint chocolate.

9. Cover the tin with a cling film.

10. Chill the marquise in the fridge for two hours.

11. Remove the marquise from the tin by using a sharp knife.

12. Serve by cutting into slices.

Lemon Syllabub

Total Prep & Cooking Time: Fifteen minutes

Yields: Four servings

Nutrition Facts: Calories: 328 | Protein: 2.2g | Carbs: 14.6g | Fat: 28.6g | Fiber: 0.2g

Ingredients:

- Two cups of whipping cream
- Half cup of caster sugar
- Three tbsps. of white wine
- Half a lemon (juice and zest)
- Berries (for serving)

Method:

1. Mix sugar and whipping cream in a bowl. Whip until soft peaks are formed.

2. Add white wine in the mixture. Mix well. Add lemon juice and lemon zest in the mixture. Combine the ingredients properly.

3. Spoon the mixture into serving bowls or glasses.

4. Sprinkle remaining lemon zest from the top.

5. Serve the lemon syllabub with berries.

Note: You can use a mix of berries or only one type of berry.

CPSIA information can be obtained
at www.ICGtesting.com
Printed in the USA
LVHW051716181020
669109LV00035B/1375

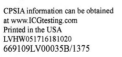

9 789814 950756